The
Insulin Resistance
Diet

*How to Stop Insulin Resistance From
Making You Fat and Ruining Your
Health*

Martin D. Kaiser, M.D.

Published By:

Dana Publishing
P.O. Box 1801
Mentor, Ohio 44060

Legal & Disclaimer

The information contained in this book and its contents is not designed to replace or take the place of any form of medical or professional advice; and is not meant to replace the need for independent medical, financial, legal or other professional advice or services, as may be required. The content and information in this book has been provided for educational and entertainment purposes only.

The content and information contained in this book has been compiled from sources deemed reliable, and it is accurate to the best of the Author's knowledge, information and belief. However, the Author cannot guarantee its accuracy and validity and cannot be held liable for any errors and/or omissions. Further, changes are periodically made to this book as and when needed. Where appropriate and/or necessary, you must consult a professional (including but not limited to your doctor, attorney, financial advisor or such other professional advisor) before using any of the suggested remedies, techniques, or information in this book.

Upon using the contents and information contained in this book, you agree to hold harmless the Author from and against any damages, costs, and expenses, including any legal fees potentially resulting from the application of any of the information provided by this book. This disclaimer applies to any loss, damages or injury caused by the use and application, whether directly or indirectly, of any advice or information presented, whether for breach of contract, tort, negligence, personal injury, criminal intent, or under any other cause of action.

You agree to accept all risks of using the information presented inside this book.

You agree that by continuing to read this book, where appropriate and/or necessary, you shall consult a professional (including but not limited to your doctor, attorney, or financial advisor or such other advisor as needed) before using any of the suggested remedies, techniques, or information in this book.

Table of Contents

Introduction

As a growing national concern, typically insulin resistance ultimately progresses to diabetes if gone unchecked. Most resources implicate that it affects 18 to 21 million Americans, and still 5 to 6 million people are not aware of it yet. That's why learning about it is the first step toward reversal. It has been revealed that diabetes is the sixth leading cause of death in the United States, with one and a half million people diagnosed each year.

Researchers account obesity and an inactive lifestyle to these figures. While these factors definitely contribute to diabetes, you will come to be aware of the underlying influences that pioneering doctors and researchers are discovering as they learn more about just how the body works.

This book contains proven steps and strategies on how to identify the signs and symptoms of insulin resistance, source the cause of the issue, and monitor your blood sugar to keep your levels within a normal range. With a dedicated effort, these proven strategies can help you or a loved one move forward from the wakeup call that has brought you to this crossroads.

This book will provide you with the basics of blood sugar maintenance, encompassing full-scale diet and exercise layouts, just to give you an idea. You will also find palliative info about still basic yet less obvious influences on reversing insulin resistance. Such examples include the importance of quality sleep, the depth and magnitude of stress factors, water intake and effective natural supplements; all ultimately mapping out a comprehensive understanding of how we are put together as dynamic living beings.

It boils down to a clear and thorough regimen of living life in a way that helps you feel your best by your own efforts. Deep down we all know what personally works for us and what doesn't when we listen to our bodies and that inner conscience that wants the best for us. Oftentimes external guidance, like road signs on the path of life, helps to direct and redirect us toward those well-intentioned goals in the midst of unfamiliar territory.

Your exploration of this topic has brought your search here for a reason. Whether recognizing the need for a change in yours or someone else's life, simply looking for more proactive information about insulin resistance or otherwise, it is a sign. This book has been written to provide you with the key facts and identifiers you need to know, supplemental information and relevant tips that perhaps you are not aware of yet regarding Insulin Resistance and how to depress it with diet and foods.

Chapter 1: What is Insulin Resistance?

Let's start with the underlying issue; Insulin, a natural regulating hormone in the body, is produced by specialized cells in the pancreas known as 'beta cells'. It promotes tissue cells in the body (muscles, skin, organs, etc.) to uptake glucose, a broken-down form of what we know as sugar, so that they may use it for energy to keep functioning properly. A side job of insulin is to help remove fat from blood and usher it into fat storage cells.

Now comparatively, while nerve cells and their impulses transmit feedback information within the body to the brain instantly, hormone feedback takes much longer because it is carried through bloodwork. That means that hormone regulation is a slow process that produces traceable results within a matter of hours while significant medical testing looks at reliable figures over weeks and months.

The common index that doctors use to determine if a person is insulin resistant is called 'A1c'. A person's A1C looks at average hemoglobin or blood sugar levels from the past three months prior to bloodwork tests. A healthy person's A1C index number should register between 4% and 5.9%, while anything at 8% or more glucose in the blood suggests insulin resistance.

Insulin Resistance

So what does being 'insulin resistant 'imply? Synonymous with the term diabetes, it reveals that glucose and fats build up in the bloodstream either because the beta cells of the pancreas decrease or cease insulin production altogether, insulin receptors in the tissue cells of the body develop a resistance to accepting the hormone, or both.

When this happens a host of issues occur. Blood sugar levels rise, stimulating further insulin production (the body's normal reaction); in the case of insulin resistance, some beta cells are still functioning and tissue cell receptors are inhibited. This leads to hyperglycemia (too much sugar in the blood) and hyperinsulinemia (excessive insulin levels in the blood) at the same time, which introduces the body to the onset of type 2 diabetes.

Further disorders result from the above situation such as an increased risk of heart disease, overloaded abdominal fat cells, and dysfunction or failure of other organs like the kidneys, bladder and liver. Abdominal fat cells function differently than what we think of in terms of fat: metabolically (converting glucose and other sources into energy), they produce several chemicals that have hostile effects on body functions. Along with that, the accumulation of blood sugars breaks down cell function, bathing the surrounding tissues.

Consider the kidneys, our vital organs that filter the blood, which become overtaxed; the bladder, which disposes the excess waste of the body and in an untreated diabetic person can show traceable amounts of sugar content; the liver, another vital organ that plays jack of all trades in terms of functional purposes, including the breakdown of red blood cells at the end of their lifetime. A crucial role of the liver recycles some of the red blood cells' components, such as the structure that provides the ability to carry oxygen to every cell of the body. We will cover further adverse effects of untreated insulin resistance later on. First, we will explore the two main varieties of diabetes that are commonly seen.

Like heart disease, insulin resistance is often a silent disorder, so it is difficult to know if one has it unless they are tested. This can be done a few ways: one way to identify it is by testing blood glucose and/or insulin after fasting when these levels should be low. A more direct test used by other specialists measures blood glucose two hours after a person consumes 75 mg or roughly one-fifth of a teaspoon of sugar. Again, a healthy person should be unaffected by this dose and present a hemoglobin range of anywhere from 80 to 110, while an insulin resistant person will test a higher number. This test is more significant for catching the disorder early on.

Type 1 Diabetes

The onset of diabetes is usually seen as either type 1 or type 2, accounting for 98% of diagnoses. Type 1 diabetes is an autoimmune disorder, developing from any number of triggers including certain drugs and chemicals, some types of infections, and a family history of the condition. It is labeled as 'autoimmune' because immune cells of the body specifically attack beta cells. Currently in mainstream medicine there is no cure for this type, leading to lifelong insulin deficiency and dependence externally. That makes it considerably more serious than type 2 diabetes however it is rare as well.

Type 1 usually reveals symptoms before the age of 30, so it is easier to catch and start receiving treatment early on in life. Because the beta cells have been killed off by the immune system, it becomes a daily responsibility to closely monitor one's activities which reduce blood sugars, their diet which can raise blood sugars at every bite, and the self-administered insulin doses to keep these levels in check. The body will have no ability to self-regulate, so with type 1 blood levels can fluctuate in extremes when not in careful check: polarities include levels high enough to cause ketoacidosis and diabetic coma to low enough that they lead to epileptic seizures from insulin shock.

Type 2 Diabetes

This is the most common form of diabetes, largely developing within people who become obese or lead relatively inactive lifestyles. In fact, roughly 90% of people with this type are overweight when diagnosed. The good news about this type is that in most cases, many who get it will see symptoms disappear and the disorder reverse itself by losing weight to reach normal BMI levels.

Exactly how this type of insulin resistance comes about currently remains a mystery because it depends on the individual. *Some develop it because of a high-carbohydrate diet that eventually wears down pancreatic function.* Others may have normal insulin production but the glucose influx proves to be too much to handle or the cells in their body that should be receiving insulin have too few receptor sites. On the other hand, alternative risk factors include metabolic syndrome, immune system issues and increased blood clotting.

The bottom line is that there are so many factors that can weigh in results of diabetic symptoms and the disorder is still being understood while doctors' current vantage point is numbers-based, leading them to diagnose based on symptoms and blood sugars alone. There are still other factors to be considered that can lead to insulin resistance reversal as forefront medical experts are finding out when incorporating psychological and emotional aspects with bodily dysfunction.

This holistic approach sees each part intimately connected with the other and aims to get to the root of the dysfunction, going beyond simply addressing physical symptoms. As doctors are learning, oftentimes physical symptoms are the last manifestation of a medical disorder and the accumulation of stress in one's life usually ushers in a deeper understanding of the core issue where the disorder can be nipped in the bud. In this light, reversal of type 2 diabetes sees greater success with certain lifestyle changes particular to the individual.

Untreated Insulin Resistance

Emergencies to consider with insulin resistance are serious and can be deadly if not properly cared for immediately. Reviewing these will reveal a few important themes pertaining to the nature of our bodies and the environment that affects them, namely pH levels. Another theme that has briefly been mentioned before and will continue to be discussed throughout this book because of its central relevance is the issue of stress and/or emotional trauma.

Our bodies optimally function at a pH level just above neutral of 7.1, being slightly basic or alkaline, while anything below 7 is acidic on the pH scale. This is a generic, all-encompassing number since we can find different pH levels occurring within different parts of the body.

It may interest you to know that certain foods like carbohydrates and especially sugar turns the body's pH levels acidic while other foods such as vegetables, especially root vegetables, and dark leafy greens, will help to alkalize the body. Maintaining a more alkaline-based diet and environment within the body is important. It has been found that an acidic body opens the gates for bacteria, pathogens, illnesses and even cancers to potentially thrive while they cannot survive in an alkaline environment. More about this will be covered in chapter 4 on food groups.

Ketoacidosis is a medical emergency in which there is a crucial lack of insulin and glucose in the cells of type 1 diabetics and only people with type 1. The body partially converts fats into energy, emitting an acidic byproduct of that metabolism called ketones that drastically changes the pH balance of the blood. A sweet or fruity odor on the breath is one way to detect this condition. Another way is to purchase test strips that measure ketone levels in the urine. This critical condition arises from various factors such as stress, infection or trauma and can amplify to shock, coma, and death.

In type 2 diabetes, the increased concentration of sugars in the blood as a solution ratio to the water in our bodies can reach exceeding levels that result in something known as

hyperosmolality. Due to such high blood sugar levels, the body's pH levels turn gravely acidic and like ketoacidosis can result in shock, coma and death.

On the other end of the spectrum, considering that insulin resistance involves an insulin imbalance that entails both too high or too low blood sugars, the latter situation can lead up to **insulin shock**. This means there is too much insulin in the bloodstream caused by a few reasons. A diabetic person could have administered too much insulin, or such factors like a skipped meal, sudden exertion, stress, infection, or trauma cause the body to metabolize all blood sugar resources. Too much insulin means very low blood sugars, known as hypoglycemia. The symptoms to watch out for in this case are dizziness, confusion, weakness in the muscles, and tremors. This case also leads to potential coma and death if gone untreated.

Chapter 2: Be Aware of the Signs and Symptoms

Between type 1 and type 2 diabetes among the other types, you may find yourself confused as how to accurately detect the signs when insulin resistance can ultimately occur at any stage in life. Rest assured that while several factors may induce its onset and many symptoms can result from it, diabetes produces specific 'tells' that you can watch out for and consult a professional about if they appear for you or a family member.

There are three basic signs that are characteristic to the onset of all types of diabetes known as the "polys". **Polyuria** refers to frequent urination above normal that is caused by elevated blood sugar; as opposed to salt, which helps to retain water within the body, excess sugar draws water out of the body's cells and is then released in the urine. You will find that this also results in chronic dehydration, which leads right into the next 'poly'.

An important side note is that if you ever find yourself with dry mouth, diabetes or not, this is the last sign of dehydration that manifests in the body meaning that you have already been dehydrated for quite some time before this symptom showed up. It should be an indicator that you need to hydrate – that is, consume water and straight up **just water** – immediately.

Polydipsia is when there is excessive thirst that is systemically linked to the loss of water with polyuria. If you find yourself or another reaching for a beverage more often than usual, or if indeed someone makes that observation about you, it should be an indicator to consider getting checked out.

Polyphagia denotes an increase in appetite. This results because the body's cells have trouble taking on glucose derived from the breakdown of digested carbohydrates. Unfortunately, these are the most effectual form of energy for the body, and in the case of diabetes the body must then convert fat stores for fuel, and after that is gone it resorts to protein (namely muscle tissues, causing them to atrophy in due time).

Symptoms deriving from these three "polys" lead to effects experienced as chronic fatigue of the body as well as mental processes, weight loss due to polyphagia and nausea and vomiting from polydipsia.

Remember that diabetes starts out subtly and silently, and while these signs might not seem like anything serious in the moment, they are often overlooked for that reason while the illness progresses to damage other organs. Just like any other serious disorder, the earlier on that it can be caught and get treated with the proper care the better. It will mean less time and work for the body to recover and stabilize, allowing you to get back into your life the way you love to live it with hopefully a healthier approach that continues to empower the quality of your daily experiences.

Complications of Diabetic Progression

Beyond the "polys" are more serious complications stemming from the progression of insulin resistance. These are more notable and obvious physical symptoms that often give way to one seeking medical attention since the person has finally realized there is something wrong, although by this time they may be a little worse off for not catching it sooner. Listed below is an easy-to-read layout of these complications with explanations for each one.

Cardiovascular disease: Because high blood glucose levels cause an acidic change in pH, the insides of the veins and arteries and those of the heart get eaten away, damaged due to insulin resistance. Along with the associative increase of fat cells in the bloodstream, it becomes an open invitation for atherosclerosis. The complication here is that unlike the typical development of atherosclerosis within the artery walls alone, **a diabetic patient will accumulate fatty plaque throughout the body**. Stroke, hypertension (high blood pressure), and aneurysm (blood clotting and blockage of vessels) all become increased risks. This is the majority cause of death in people with diabetes at about two-thirds to three-quarters of the patient population.

Edema: meaning the swelling of some part of the body, happens because of a slow and lethargic blood in the veins. It can be found within the extremities, but the lower legs, ankles and feet of a diabetic person are usually where the swelling happens. Did you know that 70 percent of blood in the body is found in the legs at any given time? It is due to gravity as well as the fact that blood flow takes much longer in veins that return it to the heart than in arteries, which contain smooth muscle to help the blood flow out. Therefore, it greatly helps insulin resistant people with edema to keep their legs raised and resting as often as possible so that gravity works for them rather than against them.

Ulcers, gangrene and amputations: These highly undesirable effects result from an epidemic of plaque buildup throughout the entire circulatory network. Because blood flow is so drastically constrained many areas of the body, especially the furthest extremities such as the feet, our natural capacity to heal and regenerate cells becomes altogether ineffective. Even small cuts and scrapes can't heal; ingrown toenails, blisters, or pressure spots on the feet can turn into a life-threatening situation. Without blood reaching these areas, the cells can die from nutrient starvation or be at the mercy of infection and pathogens without white blood cells to fight off. This becomes a noticeable sign in the form of diabetic ulcers that are usually found on the soles of the feet where pressure is applied when standing and walking. Without care, diabetes has become the reason for about 82,000 lower extremity amputations each year.

Kidney disease: The kidneys are the filtration system for all the blood that consistently runs throughout our entire body. They are also one of the first branches of the descending aorta and thus become clogged with plaque very easily. Polyuria, the constant urination symptom of diabetes that starts with the kidneys, taxes their function by causing them to work harder and can lead up to renal failure and the need for transplants.

Impaired vision: Our eyes contain millions of very tiny capillaries, which you can see usually if you have ever missed a night's sleep or swam in a pool with too much chlorine. Diabetes will thicken these blood vessels, leaving the eyes without necessary nutrition, creating a risk of micro-aneurysms, and leaking blood and proteins into the retina. The exorbitant amount of sugar in the blood can bind to proteins in the lens of the eye causing cataracts and eventually blindness. This issue is the leading cause of new blindness in people from 20 to 70 years old in the U.S.

Neuropathy: As it has been mentioned, tissues that are bathed in a highly sugary blood become weakened, damaged and eaten away at in this acidic environment. Along with absent capillary circulation, this leads to nerve damage experienced by sensations of tingling, pain, and numbness. When neuropathy hits the central nervous system (brain, brainstem, and spinal cord), the ability to maintain blood pressure becomes unstable, as well as a number of other automated systems in the body: delayed or inefficient emptying of the stomach, diarrhea, constipation and sexual impotency. This usually occurs somewhere between 10 and 20 years after diabetes is diagnosed, so people with the illness who maintain it well from diagnosis and alter their lifestyle to attempt reversal are unlikely to reach this point.

Others: Since diabetes directly involves the circulatory system and all cells in the body interact with the blood as a necessary means of functioning, pretty much every body system becomes affected by diabetes. This is why the symptoms are so wide-ranging. The disorder is also connected to UTIs, candidiasis, birth defects, aggressive ear infections that can invade the skull, and abnormal rates of gingivitis and tooth loss.

Chapter 3 : Understanding Insulin

Insulin is a bodily hormone that is supplied by the pancreas. After you eat, the pancreas produces insulin to convert glucose into energy throughout the cells in the body. Insulin is needed in metabolism. It also helps the body store energy for future use.

Without insulin, you won't have energy. Without energy, your body will not function. Your body needs energy and without it, your cells will starve – causing hunger, fatigue and sometimes, life-threatening complications such as diabetes.

Here is a glimpse of how insulin works:

Insulin directs the cells in the body to take glucose from the bloodstream and not from other sources. While there are cells in the body that can take in glucose without insulin, majority of the cells require insulin for absorption.

Insulin regulates blood sugar levels. When the body is unable to respond to insulin or produces little amounts of insulin, diabetic symptoms may form.

Insulin helps metabolism or the breaking down of nutrients that the body takes in.

Insulin signals the liver, fat cells and muscles to store unused glucose as glycogen.

To better understand the important role of insulin, you need to know how it functions with the different systems in your body. Understanding insulin and the effect it has on your body during, before and after eating will allow you to maintain stable levels of blood sugar and stay healthy, strong and energized.

Digestive, Excretory and Endocrine Systems

Your body needs energy to function and you get that energy from the food you eat. The blood sugar levels become low before you eat. When you eat, that food goes through your digestive system – from your mouth to your esophagus to your stomach and intestines. The food is broken down into smaller nutrients so that the body can absorb it and distribute it through your bloodstream.

The pancreas – that small organ located between your spine and your stomach, is responsible for producing and releasing insulin into your bloodstream as you eat. This hormone starts the process of converting glucose into energy. The energy then is distributed to different parts of your body. That is why you not only feel satiated when you eat, you also feel strengthened and invigorated.

Proper metabolism also helps the body expel waste such as perspiration, urine, and stool. If your insulin levels are stable, your bodily systems will function well.

Additionally, regular insulin levels help the liver, fat cells and muscles store energy for future use, in the form of glucose. Hence, the liver does not have to work overtime in producing glucose and maintaining your blood sugar inside a healthy range.

Circulatory System

Insulin in the bloodstream helps distribute energy to various cells in the body including the cardiovascular and central nervous systems. The bloodstream delivers the insulin so it is important that the blood sugars are within a healthy range.

If glucose builds up in the blood, a condition referred to as hyperglycemia, nerve damage can happen. It can also cause eye and kidney problems. You will feel excessive thirst and go to the bathroom frequently when you have high blood glucose.

On the other hand, you can also experience hypoglycemia or low blood glucose. Symptoms include general fatigue, confusion and mood swings such as irritation. Sometimes, too low blood sugar can lead to unconsciousness.

Hyper- or hypoglycemia can happen when the body does not have the right amount of insulin in the bloodstream to deliver energy. The body's cells starve and will look for other sources of energy such as stored fat. Moreover, a glucose buildup can also cause ketone buildup (ketoacidosis) which is a life-threatening ailment.

Insulin at Work

The food you take in will be broken down into sugars in your digestive system. The main sugar from food is called glucose. Glucose will pass through the walls of your intestines and flow into your bloodstream. Insulin helps the cells absorb the glucose in your bloodstream and turn them to energy or store them as fat.

To stay alive and healthy, the glucose levels in your blood should neither be too high nor too low. After you eat, the blood glucose levels go up, so the insulin levels should also go up. In between meals, the blood glucose levels naturally go down and your insulin levels drop. When this happens, the glycogen or stored fat will be converted into glucose into your bloodstream for the body to use.

Insulin does not only help break down glucose to distribute energy to the body – it also stores fat, which is important for future glucose requirements. People tend to believe that insulin, then, is to blame for weight gain and obesity. But nothing is farther from the truth. Find out more in the next chapter.

Chapter 4 : Insulin and Fat Storage

Fat storage is caused by insulin, but insulin does not make you fat.

There is a popular myth that insulin causes weight gain and obesity since insulin is responsible for storing unused glucose in the liver, in the muscles, and in fat cells. But insulin is not evil.

Additionally, people blame carbohydrate intake for the influx of insulin that causes havoc and imbalance in the body.

As you have read in the previous chapter, the hormone insulin is responsible for converting glucose into energy. The digestive system breaks down the food you take in such as protein, fats, and carbohydrates into amino acids, fatty acids, and glucose. These nutrients are transported into the bloodstream for cell absorption – to use or to store. Once the task is completed, the pancreas rest and insulin levels become normal. The process repeats when you eat again.

When you think of it that way, insulin is very helpful and much needed. So what makes people think that it is responsible for making them sick or fat?

Their reason is this: insulin prevents the breakdown of fat cells. It tells the body cells to use up the energy that is present in the glucose in the bloodstream instead of burning up fat stores. And when enough glucose and fatty acids are consumed, it stimulates the body to turn the rest into body fat.

In short, their logic is that when you eat a high carb diet; your insulin levels go up, which causes you to burn less fat and store more of it which leads to you getting fatter. Conversely, when you take in a low carb diet; you will have low insulin levels and store less fat as you burn more, thus you will stay lean, generally speaking.

Sound simple but it's not.

Again, insulin does not make you fat, even if it does stimulate fat storage. Insulin allows the fat cells to absorb unburned glucose and fatty acids and they may expand, but not to the point that you will become fatter than you are. **What makes you fat is not your hormone insulin, <u>it is overeating</u>**.

The Importance of Energy Balance

You need to understand that energy balance in your body means that you have equilibrium between the amount of food you take and the amount of energy you burn on a daily basis. If you eat more than what you burn through physical activity such as exercise, the excess energy will be stored in your body as fat. This makes you gain weight. And if you do this on a regular basis, say a sedentary lifestyle, you are bound to get heavier and bigger until you become obese.

On the other hand, if your food intake is less than the amount of energy you burn daily, then your body will tap into the fat stores so it will produce needed energy. Done on a regular basis, this makes you slowly lose weight.

People need to know that the body needs a certain amount of energy – from blood glucose – in order to function and stay alive. That is why food is fuel to the body. It helps the body organs operate effectively. The brain and other vital organs are glucose hogs – they use a substantial amount of energy. When you eat, your body receives a relatively bigger amount of calories or energy, meaning your glucose levels are above what is the normal amount necessary to maintain life. The body does not throw away the excess energy; it stores it for future use.

So even if insulin is responsible for fat storage, you will only get fatter when you feed your body with more calories than it actually burns. And you don't get leaner by reducing insulin levels – it only happens when you feed your body lesser calories than you normally burn.

Your carbohydrate intake and your insulin levels are not the culprits. You will not have unwanted stored fat without excess calories and you can't reduce stored fat without restricting energy. If you want to maintain your ideal, healthy weight, you should have energy balance.

Here are other important facts about insulin that you need to know:

- Insulin does not stimulate hunger.

- Insulin actually makes you feel more satiated, not hungry.

- Insulin helps build muscle mass.

- Insulin does not directly build muscle as protein synthesis does, but it contains anti-catabolic properties that help decrease the breakdown of muscle protein. In this anabolic state, the muscles grow bigger and faster.

Protein also triggers insulin production

Eating low-carb yet high-protein food actually causes higher insulin levels to be produced compared to high-carb meals. Moreover, this kind of diet may cause more dietary fat to be stored in the body.

When you have a sedentary or inactive lifestyle, you don't burn as much energy as you feed your body, so the body will have a hard time dealing with insulin. And when your body does not respond effectively to this hormone, you can develop symptoms of type 2 diabetes and be at risk for heart diseases.

In conclusion, insulin isn't your only problem when you are overweight. It is what you eat and how you live – how much you move and exercise. Stress and some illnesses are also known to cause unnecessary weight gain. If you have diabetes, when and how you take insulin injections are also a factor.

You can fine tune your glucose and insulin levels through self-monitoring and control. You can determine how exercise and different food influence your glucose levels so you can make wise decisions regarding food intake, activity and insulin dose when necessary.

More importantly, keep in mind that you need to have that energy balance – eat well and be active. Exercising regularly and having a sensible diet will make you sensitive to insulin and live healthier and longer.

Chapter 5: Insulin and Disease

Insulin is often at the core of many different kinds of diseases. Insulin in the brain, for instance, can lead to neurological disorders. Insulin, when it is too little or too much in the body causes big problems either way.

Insulin and High Sugar Diets

You learned in the previous chapters that the food you eat is converted into sugar or glucose, and is delivered throughout your body via your bloodstream. When you consume high-sugar food, there is a tendency that sugar will float around in your blood, unused. Too much blood sugar results in serious health complications such as heart diseases, amputations, kidney problems, foot problems and even blindness.

You may not realize it but the following common meals are high sugar food that you may be eating every day. Consider eliminating them from your diet:

- White flour

- Energy bars

- Meal replacement bars

- Jell-O

- Carbonated drinks (Soda, pop)

- Fruit drinks

- White, refined sugar

- Yoghurt with fruit varieties

- Nachos

- Coffee drinks

- Biscuit and Sausage gravy

- Battered fish dinners

- Chinese entrees that are deep fried

- Purchased smoothies

- Fried chicken

- Doughnuts

- Restaurant hamburgers

- Frozen meals (Even "Lean Cuisines")

It is important to sporadically check your blood sugar levels so that you can delay or prevent any serious risks to your health.

Insulin and Diabetes Conditions

One of the most well-known diseases associated with impaired insulin levels is **diabetes mellitus.**

Diabetes happens when the body does not produce insulin than it should. There are two types of this disease: type 1 and type 2. People with type 1 diabetes will experience symptoms early on and will have to live with the condition throughout their lives, while people with type 2 diabetes develop symptoms much later.

Both types of diabetes involve problems that are associated with their insulin pathway: people with type 1 diabetes have a lack of insulin, while people with type 2 diabetes have chronically high levels of insulin.

When a person has Type 1 diabetes, his body needs insulin injections in order to compensate for the lack so that the liver will not have to produce ketones. When a person has type 2 diabetes, the body does not effectively respond to insulin or in effect, resists insulin. When this is the case, the body cannot use up blood glucose, causing the pancreas to produce more insulin than normal. However, pancreatic beta cells wear out in the process, hence, people with type 2 diabetes need regular insulin injections in order to manage and maintain blood sugar levels.

People with diabetes or high blood sugar don't have normal levels of insulin in their body, sometimes caused by genetic mutations. They need insulin therapy to do the job of the pancreas. Blood tests can help a patient with diabetes know when his glucose levels are either too low or too high, then take the appropriate type of insulin.

There are different kinds of insulin treatments: *rapid-acting, intermediate-acting, long-acting, and short-acting.*

Rapid-acting insulin will get to your bloodstream in as little as 15 minutes and stay working until four hours after intake.

Intermediate-acting insulin goes to the bloodstream within 2-4 hours, but will be effective for up to 18 hours.

Long-acting insulin can maintain glucose levels for 24 hours and will start working within 2-4 hours after intake.

Short-acting insulin will work for 6 hours and get to your bloodstream within 30 minutes.

Even with insulin injection treatments, people with diabetes need to control their intake of glucose so that they can regulate their blood sugar levels.

Compared to Type 1 diabetes, Type 2 is much more dangerous. The body rarely responds to insulin treatment which means that the subject in question must implement drastic diet changes as well as exercise so the body can fight back.

Chapter 6: Insulin and Metabolic Syndrome

Metabolic syndrome, also known as **prediabetes**, is a condition that is not as widely known and understood. It is actually so poorly characterized that many people do not interpret symptoms as problems that involve insulin. They associate it with other health problems.

Symptoms of metabolic syndrome include:

- High cholesterol in the blood

- Elevated blood pressure

- Increased circumference of waist

The main cause of prediabetes is the diminished response of particular tissues such as fat and muscle to insulin in the body. Experts cannot say if metabolic syndrome can be reversed or is treatable.

Majority of people with metabolic syndrome tend to be overweight and may have other life-threatening diseases and health conditions. A good and long-term solution is to reduce the chronic blood sugar levels and re-establish the body's sensitivity to insulin.

More Energy with Less Insulin

People think that they should eat more carbohydrates so the body can have more calories to burn for energy. But carbohydrates bring insulin levels high and insulin intensifies fat storage while decreasing the body's tendency to burn fat.

When you decrease your carbohydrate intake, you may have low insulin levels, decreased appetite, weight loss and improved lipid profiles. When your insulin levels are controlled and maintained, the fat cells are liberated – they can be burned somewhere else. When insulin levels are decreased, the fat cells are released and supply the body with sufficient energy for use.

Keep in mind that people turn out to be sedentary because they are getting fat – not the other way around. When they have the right amount of energy, they tend to be more active.

The Big Picture

You need to ensure that you have a healthy and functional body metabolism to be able to understand your capability to access fat. There are different factors but controlling insulin is probably the most helpful solution with long-term results.

Managing proper levels of insulin and sensitivity will allow your body to access stored fats and convert it to energy, reducing the health risks associated with excessive body fat.

Therefore, you need to remember the old adage: you are what you eat. What and when you eat greatly affects your blood glucose and insulin levels. To reduce the danger of diabetes and metabolic syndrome, you need to consider how your diet can prevent and control imbalance as well as sustain and maintain insulin.

Chapter 7: Are You Affected?

The tricky part about having insulin resistance is the fact that it's a silent condition. It doesn't trigger any major symptoms that may cause worry or concern in the beginning. What do I mean in the beginning? I mean in the early phases before it advances to prediabetes. There isn't a possible way to detect insulin resistance on your own, simply because it shows no clear signs, unlike diabetes when there is a list of symptoms that may convince you to do a medical checkup.

However, even though there aren't any signs that may indicate the existence of insulin resistance, doing some tests and checking your insulin sensitivity cannot hurt you. You should especially be concerned about the possible occurrence of this condition if:

- You are overweight (especially around the abdomen)

- You are older than 40

- You have high cholesterol

- You have high blood pressure

- You have PCOS (Polycystic Ovary Syndrome)

- You live a sedentary lifestyle

- You have a family history of diabetes

- You had a baby who was heavier than 9 pounds

Although in the early stages, there aren't any indications of insulin resistance, once it advances, this condition can result in:

- High blood sugar

- Fatty liver

- High blood pressure

- Acne and large face pores

- Extreme hunger and food cravings

- Swollen ankles

- Apple-shaped figure

- Skin tags

- Hair loss

Insulin resistance never happens overnight. There isn't a single thing you can do that will trigger the insulin levels to suddenly rise to that point that you will become insulin resistant. This condition happens slowly, gradually and over time. Once a person becomes affected, he/she cannot know it, unless he/she gets tested. So why don't we all? Now, that is the question of the century. Why don't doctors express concerns about this condition? Why don't they suggest these kinds of tests to the patients? Whether it is for purely economic reasons, or simply because they have been trained that way is up for a debate, and a subject for a different time and place. Be as it may, one thing is for sure. Once the blood sugar levels skyrocket, it is a little too late. Why wait for the numbers of the monitor to scare us to death? Don't wait for you to show symptoms of diabetes so that your doctor suggests a fasting blood sugar test. From time to time, checking yourself for insulin resistance will not do you any harm. In some cases, that one decision can be life-saving.

The glucose tolerance test is the most reliable test for insulin resistance. It is a test when the patient is given glucose and when blood samples are taken in order to detect the way in which the glucose is absorbed. This will indicate whether the insulin does its job properly or not. Usually, this test is done within 2 hours. First the blood glucose is checked while the patient is fasting, and then again at 1 and 2 hour intervals.

Measuring the lipid hormones can also give a pretty good insight of the fat metabolism and insulin relationship.

If your test results show insulin resistance, it doesn't mean that you are in danger, but that you have dodged a bullet, since knowing this condition before it advances into something more dangerous gives you a pretty good lead and the chance to do the right thing to reverse it.

Chapter 8: Reversing It Naturally

At this point most readers are going to realize that that the only possible way to reverse insulin resistance is through a healthy diet and balanced lifestyle.

Since the insulin is in charge of persuading muscle, liver, and fat to absorb the glucose, when there is insulin resistance they are not doing this efficiently, limiting the sugar intake is more than crucial in order to stop it from piling up in the blood which results in diabetes.

Needless to say, the solution is simple. That chocolate icing cake may put a smile on your face, but it will also kill the fat cells in your belly and will create a pouch, which let's face it, despite the fact that it will not look good in that new shirt you bought the other day, it will also increase the insulin spikes and contribute to more serious health complications.

And is there a better way to approach such a condition than with what nature has to offer? In my opinion, the natural approach is the only weapon you will ever need when fighting a war like this. People in the past didn't know of another way to treat a condition. Why do we always try to take the 'easy way out'? Why do we think that taking medications will resolve our issues? Read on to find out how to reverse insulin resistance naturally.

Beware the Culprits

The truth is, whenever your cells are exposed to insulin, they become more insulin resistant. That is an inevitable fact, and there is absolutely nothing you can do to change the course in which the process of absorbing the glucose from the bloodstream works. However, we can do a lot to help our body out. We can reverse insulin resistance and improve our overall health by paying attention to the food we ingest. By making sure that the pancreas will not get such an increased demand for producing insulin, we can move towards a much healthier life.

But where do we start? How to know what to eat and what not to eat? What food requires an increased release of insulin? Here is what should be tossed in your garbage can immediately if you want to stop this condition:

Sugar. Is it really necessary for me to explain this? It is clear as day that people with insulin resistance should purge this sweet hazard from their diets. When I say purge, I mean say goodbye to sugar for good. And no, honey is not the healthier choice, not for you anyway.

Trans Fats. If you are looking for the unhealthiest type of fats, let me introduce you to trans fats. When hydrogen is added to unsaturated fats, trans fats are born. Besides that they cause inflammation, next to sugar, they are the second enemy to your insulin sensitivity. You will mostly find this kind of fats in cans and packages.

Bad Carbs. Since there is an ongoing debate and misunderstanding regarding which type of carbs are good and which are bad, let me explain the confusion. Some may think potatoes are bad since they are carb-loaded, well this is not entirely true. You see, a single potato weighing 6 ounces it is mostly made of water; only 23% of its entire weight are carbs. On the other hand, a rice cake may weigh 1/5 ounce, but 80% of its weight is carbohydrate. The bad carbs are mostly found in bread, bagels, white rice, pasta, crackers, cereals, etc.

High-Lactose Dairy. Some may disagree with this, but it is the truth. Milk and other high-dairy products torment our tummies, making the pounds stick around our abdomen and contribute to insulin resistance. How? As any other type of food, when we ingest lactose, it is broken down by the lactase enzyme. So where is the problem? The problem is that as we grow older, our body produces less of the lactase enzyme, and it makes it hard for our bodies to digest lactose.

Gluten. Grains, such as wheat, are made of a sticky protein called gluten that is surely unfriendly, not only to your body shape but also to your health, since it is known that it can elevate the blood sugar, which you want to avoid at all costs. Gluten also leads to inflammation, which is yet another reason to keep it off your kitchen.

Soda. If you thought that you could trick your gut by satisfying your sweet tooth and drinking a sugary drink, you were wrong. Besides the obvious fact of spiking your blood sugar, you should also avoid soda because it has a huge contribution to gaining weight. Switching to diet coke is not a healthy alternative either.

Processed Meat. Processed meat may bring out some amazing flavors to your sandwich, but it is not kind to your health. It is packed with calories that will wrap your belly and contribute to insulin resistance. Besides that, it contains additives and nitrates that may cause additional health problems.

Beware the Organic Trap. These days, you can buy just about anything in 'organic' version. But just because the label says it's organic it doesn't mean that it is healthy for you. By eating organic cookies, you are adding to your belly weight and supporting insulin resistance, the same way as if you were eating regular chocolate cookies.

Your Kitchen "Must-Haves"

Just like there is a list of food that should be off limits for those trying to reverse insulin resistance and get their tissues to absorb the blood glucose the way they should, there is also a long list of foods that should be a part of their kitchen and pantry. I am talking about the healthy choices, the foods that contribute to lowering blood sugar and improving insulin sensitivities.

Having insulin resistance doesn't mean that there will be nothing but green vegetables in your fridge. In fact, you will be surprised to know about the variety of delicious foods that should be a part of your diet. Thinking that you will not enjoy cooking again? Well, think again, because you better throw these food items in the shopping cart the next time you visit the supermarket.

Omega 3 Fatty Acids. Although it is long believed that omega 3 fatty acids have the potential to somehow improve the insulin sensitivity, now it is known how. Omega 3 fatty acids interact with the cell receptors in a way that they allow them to bind more of the hormone insulin easily and therefore help reverse insulin resistance. You can find omega 3 fatty acids in cold water fish like salmon, sardines, trout, tuna, herring, oyster and flax seeds. This is excellent news for the fish lovers, but for those of you who don't eat fish, make sure to substitute it with some omega 3 fatty acid supplements, since these acids play a major role in reversing insulin resistance.

Fruits and Vegetables. Now, we all know the importance of fresh fruit and vegetables in our diet, whether we are suffering from a health condition or not. However, those who want to control and reverse their insulin resistance should make sure to follow this diet rule, since most of the studies regarding this and similar conditions have shown that eating a variety of fruits and veggies help in improving the overall health. Here is what you absolutely must have in your kitchen:

Blueberries – Thanks to their chemical called anthocyanins, blueberries stimulate the release of adiponectin, which helps the body to increase its sensitivity to insulin and lower the blood glucose.

Leafy Green Vegetables – Spinach, broccoli, kale, collard greens and other leafy greens play a major role in reversing insulin resistance and repairing damaged blood vessels. They are amazing antioxidants, rich in fiber and real vitamin bombs.

Indian Gooseberry – Also called amla fruit, Indian gooseberry is one of the most important natural cure in the Ayurvedic medicine. It promotes a proper pancreas function and boosts insulin sensitivity.

Always aim for fruits and veggies with a low glycemic index such as avocado, tomatoes, all berries, onions, citrus fruit, mushrooms, grapes, nectarines, asparagus, pears, etc.

If you cannot find some types of fruit or vegetables to buy fresh, know that the frozen ones are just as healthy.

Whole Grains. According to many studies (most of them published in the European Journal of Clinical Nutrition), implementing whole grains into your diet can contribute to reversing insulin resistance, or reducing the risk for those not affected by this condition. Barley, whole wheat, oats, bulgur, and spelt, support the managing of the blood sugar and improving the insulin sensitivity. So, throw that cereal package away and enjoy a healthy bowl of oatmeal for breakfast instead.

Nuts. Nuts, especially walnuts, should be an important part of your path to reversing insulin resistance. According to a study performed by the University of California, walnuts boost insulin sensitivity, contribute to managing the blood sugar levels, lower cholesterol and can slow down the growth of a prostate cancer.

Legumes. Legumes are known to have the power to manage the levels of glucose in the blood, but not only diabetics can benefit from adding them to their meals. People who are insulin resistant should also make lentils, peas, chickpeas and beans, especially cannelloni beans, a significant part of their diet since they can make the muscle, liver, and fat respond to insulin more effectively.

Monounsaturated Fats. Monounsaturated fats are those kinds of fats that are found in the plants. They can be found in olive oil, canola oil, walnut oil, avocados, nuts, and seeds, etc.

Nut butters are a great choice for insulin resistant people since they are monounsaturated, contribute to controlling the insulin sensitivity and can provide you with enough proteins to keep your tummy full and energize you.

Spices. If you enjoy spicing up your meals, then here are some good news for you – go ahead. There are many spices that can contribute to reversing insulin resistance.

Cinnamon – This flavorful spice increases our ability to respond to insulin, and therefore must be a part of an insulin resistance diet. There are many heavy clinical studies that have shown how cinnamon reduces the fasting blood sugar levels. If you implement less than a half a teaspoon of cinnamon each day, it will have a significant impact on your improving insulin goal.

Turmeric – The *curcumin* compound found in turmeric is a powerful antioxidant packed with anti-inflammatory properties. A study published in Molecular Nutrition & Food Research says that turmeric has an important effect in preventing problems associated with insulin resistance such as liver diseases.

Ginger, fenugreek, garlic, cayenne pepper, cumin, and ginseng are other spices that are known to help manage the blood sugar and control insulin resistance.

Herbs and Leaves. There are many herbs, leaves and leave extracts that can contribute to improving your health by managing the insulin and blood sugar levels.

Mango Leaves – Used for centuries as a remedy in Chinese medicine, mango leaves are a great addition to your diet, since they can help you regulate the insulin and control the blood glucose levels. And implementing mango leaves in your diet couldn't be simpler; just boil 2-3 leaves in a cup of water, drink the tea warm, and enjoy.

Spirulina – Although not so much an herb, actually an acyanobacteria, spirulina is a blueish green algae that is safe to consume. You can find it in a powder form in most well-equipped health stores. Research shows that spirulina can improve insulin sensitivity by an incredible 225%.

Green Tea. Many studies have shown that the antioxidant called epigallocatechin gallate that can be found in green tea can promote proper insulin activity and keep the blood sugar levels in check.

Olive Leaf Extract. A research performed by the University of Aukland has found that the extract from the olive leaves can nudge the pancreas to increase its production of insulin, which can clearly contribute to controlling and eventually reversing the insulin resistance.

Natural Supplements

If you are against drugs (and you should be, unless of course, your condition requires some serious treatment) you can talk to your physician about the alternative of adding natural supplements to your diet.

Magnesium. People that are insulin resistant are usually deprived of this essential nutrient. Magnesium is known to regulate the insulin sensitivity and contribute to managing the blood sugar.

Vanadium. If you are looking for a mineral that will surely optimize the glucose tolerance, then that's vanadium. Vanadium works in an almost exact way as the insulin, and that is why it is said that it mimics it. Studies have shown that vanadium can increase the insulin sensitivity and decrease the body fat and the appetite at the same time.

Chromium. One of the essential minerals that can enhance the activity of the insulin and lower the risk of cardiovascular diseases. Although it is normal for our cells to be more deficient of this mineral as we grow old, it is proven that people with insulin resistance and type 2 diabetes have significantly lower chromium levels than those who are not affected by these conditions. Talk to your doctor and see if there is a need for you to take a chromium supplement.

Berberine. Berberine is a compound that can be found in the roots of some plants such as Oregon grape, barberry, and goldenseal. Its association with insulin resistance is simple. Berberine can lower the blood sugar and decrease the demand for insulin production, which can improve insulin sensitivity. People suffering from diabetes are encouraged to take berberine supplement since there are many studies that have found that this beneficial compound can actually be as effective as diabetes drugs, without the possible side effects, of course.

Garcinia Cambogia. Although it is primarily a weight-loss aid since it decreases the hunger, diabetics and people who are insulin resistant can indeed benefit from supplementing their diet with Garcinia Cambogia. The hydroxycitric acid that Garcinia Cambogia contains can delay the absorption of the blood glucose levels after meals, which can clearly improve the glucose metabolism. This acid orders the liver to store more glucose levels than the fat.

Chapter 9: Take a Stand

Would you or someone you know rather cope with insulin resistant, or would you like to take proactive steps in keeping those levels steady and progressively stabilizing?

Exercise and physical exertion have their place in the recovery regimen; however in the practice of monitoring blood glucose levels, it is crucial to know that any mild to strenuous activity is going to cause those levels to drop. Know where your levels are before engaging in such activities in order to avoid them dropping too low and risking insulin shock.

The fact is there are other significant ways to lose weight that are equally if not more effective than exercise. This is important to know in the case of people with type 2 diabetes, especially if the weight gain has caused them to become obese and onset the disorder in the first place. Many overweight people have found that with a shift in their diet alone, they were dropping pounds faster than cardio or working out. Food helped create the problem, and likewise, it can be the solution. The emphasis is on **what kinds of foods your body responds well to** and **portion size**. Everybody is different; results are not the same for everyone. You have to test.

Proper nutrition ensures that we are providing the body with its needs rather than its wants and cravings and within volumes that it is capable of handling. Providing the right portions at mealtimes will train the body to regulate itself again; not have to work as hard at digestion, whose ability and quality to process food is a major determiner of our overall health; and get the most out of what we feed ourselves with no great expenditure on waste production. Symptoms like acid indigestion, gassiness and bloating will phase out, and any foul odors produced by the body (commonly traced to sugar and stress caused by various reasons) will become neutralized.

This process indeed will take time and a fair amount of discipline to see it through but it does not have to be a struggle. On the contrary, within the first week, you will begin noticing results from an overall improvement in mood to the reduction and relief of some physical symptoms, as well as feeling **good** in your body. Essentially you will be treating your body with what it **needs** and it will be thanking you for it.

Many people who have changed up their diet to appropriately suit their body's needs have experienced weight loss quickly.

A psychological study was conducted in the early 2000's on hotel maids, many of whom were overweight, pertaining to weight loss and the awareness of the activities they did in their work. They were interviewed and monitored individually and their daily home, work, and eating habits were all documented.

Then the focus group of maids was divided in two, group A and group B. Group B was left as a control group to continue with their tasks unaltered by the study. Group A, however, was presented information so rudimentary that it is mesmerizing how deeply it affected them to produce the results that were observed. It unveiled certain truths about how dynamically we are put together that can and will be studied for decades to come.

Group A was told not to change any of their eating or home habits for the next few months, which across the board were mildly active to relatively sedentary outside of their work. The group was then questioned and presented with the information by the researchers, asking the maids if they were aware that the work they were doing in the hotels was actually exercise. Most all of them answered 'no'. Basic tasks like emptying garbage pails, changing bed sheets, cleaning bathrooms and vacuuming rooms were just considered to be part of the job.

The researchers then presented the group with an outline of how many calories each task burned within the body as they were performed and asked the maids to keep this in mind while they were working for the next few months. Ultimately, after this course of time most all of the maids were observed to experience some amount of weight loss, from a few pounds up to 20 pounds. Group B, on the other hand, had not seen much of any changes in their weight.

The maids in group A had not gone to the gym or changed their lifestyle except for an increase in the awareness of their actions and the effect it has on the body. This example has been brought to you to illustrate an important concept that will greatly accelerate your healing process and overall quality of life, which also pertains to the laws of attraction. The mind tells the body what to do both consciously and unconsciously, and with practice and awareness, we can learn to control our thoughts to create a new state of living for ourselves.

Controlling and reversing insulin resistance starts with nutrition. Changing the diet to incorporate nourishing foods for the body will help to change its internal environment that will, in turn, promote gradual weight loss. It will also prime the body and the mind to relax into a healthier state that makes the ensuing recovery process all the easier. Who knows, you or a loved one might just find yourselves having FUN with it, knowing that you are healing, taking back control of your life, and doing more to feel great about yourselves.

As for exercise, let's reiterate that vigorous activity only puts more strain on the body. That is not what a recovering body needs to improve health when the organs are already taxed and the potential of plaque buildup in the veins and arteries is present. This form of exercise we're talking about, which tends to be a common concept, raises the heart rate and blood circulation and causes the other organs such as the kidneys, lungs and liver to work harder. Not to say that cardio, aerobics, and weight training have their place down the road to recovery, and suggestions will be detailed in chapter 5, however, there are milder forms of activity to stimulate the body and meet its needs in a weakened state.

These exercises are characteristically slow, calm and controlled, so each repetition brings about mindfulness.

When we move slowly, we can focus more closely on performing the specific action with regard to good body mechanics, in turn promoting body awareness. Better body awareness prevents strain in motion and promotes better posture which removes strain on the muscles, internal organs, joints, and nerves.

This subsequently removes any stress on the mind; feeling good in the body means feeling good in the mind and more relaxed. As we relax with these slow exercises, we open up the blood flow in a healthy way to increase circulation. By synchronizing our breath with the movement, we are actively and consciously nurturing the blood and therefore the rest of the body, including the mind, with fresh oxygen. Filling the body with oxygen encourages the cells to relax more deeply and function properly. The reason illness is referred to as a "dis-ease" is because the basic problem has stemmed from some sort of stress that has brought us out of a relaxed state of being over time and consistency.

To sum up, slow, controlled exercises with synchronized breathing promote the body and mind with relief. They reduce stress and physical strain and create a more prominent environment for the body to heal, as is its natural ability. These types of exercises connect the mind and body to form a healthy relationship with each other, listen to each other's true needs, and work as one to allow you to focus on and live out your true desires and goals. As with anything worth doing and getting better at, it may not feel like much at first but with paced practice and consistency the results will speak for themselves. The key point here is that you do not need to do hard core training, weight lifting or cardio to achieve results with a switched diet, sometimes the body will respond much better to slow relaxed work outs; such as maybe a 2-3 mile fast walk in the park everyday.

Weight gain is related to a number of reasons, however, most can be traced back to the types of foods we eat, the portions, how active we are day to day, as well as how much stress we take on and **hold on** to. Think about how often you reach for fatty, salty, and/or sugary foods when you need comfort or relief.

Think about, and really take the time to shed some awareness on this, the thoughts and mood we're absorbed in while we eat. Do we eat fast just to get something in our bodies, or do we take the time to really enjoy the meal and each bite?

Chapter 10: The Nutrition Connection

In our modern world more and more people are overfed and undernourished. The empty calories eaten by so many should not even be considered food. If you have started to go down the slippery slide that leads to obesity, you are among millions of others. If you do your part to support your body, there is a road leading back to health. But don't expect instant results, after all it took time to get to where you are now, and it will take time to get back up that slope. Nutrition can go a long way to heal your metabolism, balance your blood sugar level, improve your body composition, and make you feel energized. First, and foremost you must make a commitment to always choose real, whole foods. (And no, that does not mean eating a whole donut) You must also learn how to combine these foods to give you a steady supply of energy and nutrients.

The difference between GI (glycemic index) and GL (glycemic load)

The glycemic index measures how rapidly the carbohydrate in a given food turns into sugar. Glucose is given the value of 100, and the higher the GI of a food, the higher the blood sugar spike it creates. The more accurate measure is the glycemic load (GI divided by 100 and multiplied by the foods carbohydrate content) because it takes the fibre content of the food into consideration.

Here are some examples:

- Shredded Wheat Cereal - GI: 69, GL: 57
- Cornflakes - GI: 84, GL: 72.7
- Carrots - GI: 71, GL: 7.2
- Sweet potato - GI: 54, GL: 13.1

So a food with a high glycemic index is not necessarily bad for you, look at the glycemic load instead. Carrots are a good example to demonstrate this. But remember, if you juice carrots, you are getting rid of the fiber. Carrot juice will have a high glycemic load.

In general foods that are refined, processed or contain a lot of sugar while lacking in protein, fats and fiber will have higher glycemic loads. And basically this is all you need to remember. Avoid refined processed foods. Combine healthy, whole protein, fat, and fiber with your carbs at each meal, and you will be on the road to healing. Example, sweet potatoes and vegetables with some nuts on the side, or a large bowl of natural oatmeal missed with blueberries and almonds.

What you Need to Know about Food Groups

You may be familiar with Health Canada's Food Guide, or the new American food guide, Choose My Plate. These have come a long way since the food guides were first published, but on closer inspection, they still have many recommendations that are not health promoting. Some items that you should not eat that are included in Canada's Food Guide are margarine, canola oil, mayonnaise (this latter is fine if it is home made from fresh ingredients, but somehow I doubt that is what they meant). Margarine is not a real food, it is highly processed, treated with all sorts of chemicals, and void of nutrients, so whether hard or soft you should avoid it. The American guide lists these same unhealthy oils and cottonseed oil as well. So instead of following any food guide, learn about real, whole foods, and use them to regain your health.

Protein

Protein is needed for building muscle, repairing tissue, making hormones. It keeps you feeling full and satisfied longer, and reduces cravings. From our perspective it is important, because it helps balance blood sugar, and mood. You have to make sure you get enough, but not too much. As a general guideline, at each meal you should eat protein that is approximately the size of the palm of your hand. When choosing protein sources try to include a wide variety. Always choose organic, preferably grass fed beef or lamb, and pasture raised chicken or turkey, wild caught fish.

Vegetarian sources include legumes, nuts peas and seeds. These have to be combined to make sure they provide all the essential amino acid. Combining two or three of them usually gives you the quantity of protein you need.

Fats

Fats have been given a bad reputation, but in reality are just as essential for our health as proteins are. All of our cells need fats; they are components of the cell membrane. Fats fuel the nervous system, lubricate joints, and how would you absorb fat soluble vitamins, such as vitamin A, E, and D without fat? It is important to know your fats though. The title of the book on fats, written by Udo Erasmus, says it all: **Fats that Heal, Fats that Kill**.

You do not want anything to do with trans fats, and in order to avoid them, you need to stay away from most commercial baked goods. (But you are going to avoid these anyway, since they are heavily processed, void of nutrients, and full of simple carbs.)

The fact that trans fats are unhealthy probably did not come as a surprise, but did you know that polyunsaturated fats (PUFAs) can also be dangerous. Here we have to make a distinction though, vegetable oils are generally unhealthy, oils form nuts and seeds, if properly prepared can be healthy. Vegetable oils usually come from corn, soy, or canola — three crops that are very often genetically modified. These plants are then processed beyond recognition. Since PUFAs are very unstable, the food industry uses all sorts of horrible chemicals to deodorize and preserve vegetable oils. Unfortunately the fate of sunflower and sesame oils, which are also PUFAs, is similar. Processing makes them lifeless, and downright harmful.

Then there are the healthy PUFAs coming from nuts and seeds. They are unrefined, cold pressed, not subjected to oxidative damage or chemical processing. They are stored in opaque bottles to protect them from light. Each one has a unique color and a unique taste. These you can, and should enjoy. Once the bottle is opened, keep it in the fridge. Have you ever tasted walnut oil or pumpkinseed oil on your salad? They are delicious, so try them. But remember, these oils can go rancid quickly and should not be exposed to heat. Never cook with them.

You need to get your essential fatty acids (EFAs), which are omega-6s and omega-3s, from your diet. Your body cannot synthetize them form other fats, and they are essential for good health. Every single cell needs omega-3s to keep the cell membrane flexible. The ratio of omega-6s to omega-3s in our dict should be 2:1. Since omega 3s are the ones lacking in most cases, taking a high quality omega-3 supplement is a good idea. Food sources of omega-3 include cold water fish such as mackerel, sardines, herring, and wild-caught salmon.

Saturated fats are natural, stable, and they do not oxidize. They are safe and healthy. I know, this goes against what you have been hearing for decades, but saturated fats are the best for cooking and baking. They can stand heat without oxidizing. We have seen that omega-3s make the cell membrane flexible; saturated fats add structure and stability to the cell membrane. This, however, is not their only function. They help protect the lining of the intestinal tract. They are needed for calcium absorption, for hormone production, and for the proper function of a variety of other organs.

Carbohydrates

Carbs are bad for you, right? The answer is a resounding no. Glucose is needed by your cells to produce energy. But too much of a good thing can be a problem. Staying healthy is all about balance. And again, as with fats, not all carbs are created equal. Complex carbohydrates take a lot longer for your digestive system to break down, so the sugar from them is released into you bloodstream at a much slower rate. Simple carbohydrates on the other hand enter into your bloodstream almost immediately.

Refined and processed carbohydrates are the worst offenders, they spike your blood sugar, and the resulting fall spells disaster for your waistline and for your health. Listing them all here is an impossible mission, but here are some examples for you: fruit juice, donuts, muffins, cookies and cakes, white bread (and all related baked products, such as buns, baguette, croissants, pitas), pasta, white rice, all-purpose flour, and white sugar. You get the picture?

Eat a moderate amount of complex carbohydrates, along with protein, a healthy fat, and fiber, to further slowdown their absorption and you will be fine. Complex carbohydrates include vegetables, peas, beans, lentils and whole grains.

Another distinction that has to be made is the difference between glucose and fructose. Fructose, in its natural form, found in fruits, is OK in moderation, but the highly processed high fructose corn syrup, which gets metabolized in a totally different way from glucose, is truly a poison. Over time it damages the liver, while all along it makes you crave more food, and thus contributes to weight gain. More information on this can be found in the lecture entitled **Sugar: The Bitter Truth** by Robert H. Lustig, M.D. (UCSF Division of Endocrinology and Metabolism).

In Praise of Vegetables

Veggies come in all shapes and sizes, but they all contain lots of vitamins, minerals, and phytonutrients. We have been told over and over: "Eat you fruits and vegetables!" What you should be telling yourself instead is: "Eat your vegetables and fruits" The emphasis should be on veggies, and an array of colorful ones at that.

Fruits are full of nutrients and antioxidants for sure, but they are high in simple carbs, and can easily spike your blood sugar levels. (Of course they are not all created equal, some of them, like bananas and mangoes have a higher concentration of sugar, than let´s say berries.)

Your goal should be to gradually increase your intake of vegetables until you reach 8 to 10 half cup servings per day. Focus on non-starchy vegetables (starchy ones tend to increase your blood sugar level). Here are some examples to choose from: celery, peppers, zucchini, broccoli, cauliflower, leafy greens, tomatoes, fennel.

Heard the Expression "Eat the Rainbow"?

Ever wondered why? Your body needs many nutrients in order to be able to efficiently regulate the conversion of glucose into energy. Nutrient deficiency can influence how well your body can control blood sugar levels and thus can contribute to insulin resistance. Eating a wide variety of colorful veggies and fruits can help maintain healthy vitamin and mineral levels. They all have their own, individual benefits as well.

Here are what the different colors can do for you:

Red foods contain lycopene, a phytochemical that helps prevent prostate cancer, and sun damage on the skin

Orange foods are high in carotenoids that are helpful in preventing cancer (they repair damaged DNA). Beta-carotene, also called pro-vitamin A, is important for the eyes.

Yellow foods are also beneficial to the eyes. They contain lutein and zeaxanthin, nutrients known for reducing the risk of macular degeneration and cataracts.

Green foods are high in minerals and B vitamins, greens are beneficial to the circulatory system, and are also important in cancer prevention.

Purple and blue foods are high in antioxidants, help circulation thereby protecting against heart problems.

White foods, such as onions, garlic and leeks contain allicin, which is an anti-viral, anti-fungal, anti-bacterial compound.

Chapter 11: Foods that Encourage Insulin Resistance

You have to be very careful when you eat if you are suffering from insulin resistance. Any bad choices you make will make your situation worse – sometimes dramatically so if you are not careful and start downing glasses of juice unaware of their high-sugar content.

Insulin resistance can only be only be overcome with patience and by disciplining yourself. We shall now look at some foods that are really bad choices when it comes to reducing insulin resistance and things that should be avoided where possible.

Candy or confectionary

Now this is pretty obvious. Any type of candy you eat is harmful for you as it involves direct refined sugar intake. The sugar we eat is produced after sugarcane is chopped up, boiled, crystallized and then the healthier brown sugar is stripped leaving only white sugar which is then blitzed up to make it more powdered.

At this highly refined level you are putting almost straight glucose into your body. There is very little digestion involved when you eat the refined sugars found in candy and too much can cause insulin resistance in people with even a relatively healthy weight (which is why soda is so dangerous).

Candy not only raises the sugar level in blood, but they also create further complications for insulin resistant people.

If you want to eat something sweet, eat fruit or yogurt because the sugars in those foods take longer to process and give a slower release of glucose.

Avoid candies at all costs. The question about whether to avoid sugar-free candy if possible is a touchy one, as some sources indicate artificial sugars can induce similar reactions to actual sugar, but without the same source of energy.

Studies carried out on mice at the **Weizmann Institute of Science** hinted that some sweeteners such as saccharin might change the balance of your gut and how you process glucose. Saccharin is actually not used as much in diet drinks or sugar-free candy any longer and the study used very high quantities, but it's not clear what the story is with sweeteners.

It's almost certain that they are nowhere near as bad as regular sugar and with so much invested in sweeteners people are careful about making negative claims. For many people sweeteners are a good way of enjoying foods they enjoy without endangering their health so it's up to you to make a decision.

If you think the benefits of diet drinks and sweets are worth it (because they will help you lower your sugar intake) then consider having them in moderation.

Fruit juices

Although fruits are a very healthy option to eat for people who have insulin resistance, it is important to know that fruit juices are not.

Even freshly made juices are not so good (even without added sugar there is still plenty of sugar), and neither is the 100% fruit juice that is available in the market as they all contain high levels of sugar.

Some fruit juice (such as cranberry juice) have more sugar in it than a soda drink and if you go for the smoothie variety you are losing a lot of the fiber that helps slow digestion.

This is simply because you are consuming many pieces of fruit at once. You can some fruits on a low-carbohydrate diet, but you cannot drink it in liquid form.

Some flavored waters may give you the juice hit and vegetable juices are usually relatively low in sugar (if you want to drink a cup of raw carrot and spinach that is). Ice tea or cucumber or lemon water may even hit the spot. Always make sure to check the sugar content of these drinks though.

Raisins and dried Fruits

While many types of nuts are good for insulin resistant people, raisins are not as they can be harder to digest than grapes and you can be tempted to eat a lot and consume a lot of condensed sugar.

Other dried fruits like dates or figs can be surprisingly bad for digestion and often come candied, so be careful if you choose to indulge. The drying process often saps a fruit of anything but it sugar.

When you get a handful of raisin imagine that each one is a grape. Would you have just eaten six grapes at once otherwise?

Pancakes or waffles

Pancakes and other sweet treats are among the worst breakfast choice that an insulin resistant person can make. Both pancakes and syrup contain a lot of carbohydrates and cause a lot of problems in your blood sugar levels.

When you have a craving for pancakes or waffles, suppress it, and instead make an egg with vegetables or low-GI toast. Or alternatively consider making a healthier pancake with sweet potato and use a lower-sugar topping like berries, cinnamon, etc.

French fries and other fried foods

Potatoes contain a lot of starch, when you fry them in oil, you are making it even worse for yourself.

Uncooked starchy foods are basically inedible (or are difficult to digest) so they are not really a great source of energy if you are looking to lower blood sugar.

Potatoes can also absorb a lot of oil and hence you are eating a lot of fat and extra calories if you eat fried potatoes. Eating French fries can lead to more problems associated with insulin resistance.

In general fried foods are terrible for your health; they are covered in refined carbohydrates and fried in the worst fats possible. It's not really possible to fry in healthier oils because they don't always work as well at higher heats and they are expensive to use in such large quantities.

If you do crave fried foods or French fries then consider opting for a healthy alternative. You can make your own fries by baking slice up potatoes with a little oil in the oven and you can turn to egg whites and wholegrain breadcrumbs in the oven to make a relatively healthier type of 'fried' chicken.

White bread and refined foods

White bread is a type of refined starch and it acts almost like pure sugar when it goes into your body. White bread is a really bad choice when it comes to insulin resistance.

Do not eat white bread at all if you can avoid it. Choose whole wheat bread instead which is usually brown in color.

In general white rice, bread, or pasta (or anything that is a refined carbohydrate) are the worst options and you should always opt for a whole wheat or wholegrain alternative.

Many people will find that the slightly malty taste is preferable and your blood sugar levels will thank you in the end.

Whole milk and dairy products

We discussed in the good food section that milk is good for insulin resistant people. But it is to be kept in mind that whole milk contains a lot of fat, which is not good for insulin resistance.

Many dairy products like cheese and butter are sources of saturated fats which may be worse for your cholesterol and some argue that digesting them is harder on the insulin in your body. Some doubt this and say dairy products and animal fats might be quite a good choice over some alternatives as they have some vital nutrients in them and can actually be lower in calories.

You should nevertheless choose low-fat milk or skimmed milk when considering your options. Low-fat milk in fact is a great food for insulin resistant people for the reasons outlined above, but should be had in moderation.

Bacon and processed meat

Bacon and other meats like it are very high fat meats. It has a lot of health disadvantages and should be avoided for the most part, even by otherwise healthy individuals.

Recent studies even suggest it is carcinogenic and it will put you at higher risk of cancer if you it too much too regularly.

As people with insulin resistance have a greater chance of heart diseases, bacon and other high-fat meats can be almost like poison because they make you fat very quickly.

Leaner bacon with the rind cut off might be okay as a treat, but never as anything more. Since meat can be a good source of protein you don't want to get rid of the role that bacon fill so consider replacing it with slices of lean turkey or ham – most supermarkets will have varieties that hit the spot without hurting your health.

Cakes, Pastries and Snacks

Most sweet snacks, cakes and pastries are full of sugar and should be avoided at all costs. They create spikes in blood sugar level and can cause inflammation in certain parts of the body.

Insulin cannot act properly when you eat these foods, and for people who have insulin resistance this means big problems. Don't be fooled by the branding of homemade produces either; sometimes homemade foods can actually have higher levels of sugar because nobody is regulating what goes in.

If you really love your pastries and cakes you can make your own with a lot of reduced sugar, but keep this being a treat for yourself and always use wholegrain flours and sugars if possible. Many recipes can have the sugar content severely reduced or replaced with chunks of fruit like apples.

Chapter 12: Cleanse and Detoxify

Feeling out of sync or sluggish? Are you in constant battle with fatigue, skin breakouts, aches, unexplainable pains and digestive problems and not forgetting, a constant struggle with weight loss? Well, your body is placing a distress call and it's about time for a great detox.

This is the first thing you should do before embarking on an Insulin Resistance Diet. For faster health and weight loss results, you should first cleanse your system.

As with all the principles of the Insulin Resistance Diet, we are going to do the detox au natural. By removing and eliminating all toxins from your body and feeding on a fresh, natural and wholesome diet, you will not only protect your body from disease but you will also renew your ability to attain optimum health and set yourself up for successful and sustainable weight loss.

Cleansing and detoxifying naturally

Basically, cleansing and detoxifications means cleaning your blood. This is achieved by removing impurities and free radicals from the blood in your liver, where toxins are usually processed for elimination. Your body also eliminates toxins through your intestines, kidneys, lymph's, lungs and skin.

However, when your body is compromised, impurities are not filtered in the right way and every cell in your body is adversely affected.

A healthy detox program helps your body's natural cleansing process by:

- Stimulating your liver to eliminate toxins from your body
- Resting your organs through periodic fasting
- Improving your blood circulation
- Promoting elimination of toxins through your kidneys, intestines and skin; and
- Rejuvenating your body with healthy negative calorie foods

The reason natural detoxification works is because it addresses the specific needs of individual cells which are the smallest units of human life.

How do you know that your body needs detoxification?

Today, with more toxins in our environment than ever before, it's essential to detox in order to keep our bodies functioning smoothly. We recommend that you detox your body at least once a year. You know that you need to detox if you experience symptoms such as:

- Allergies
- Unexplained fatigue
- Regular bloating
- Menstrual irregularities
- Sluggish elimination
- Mental confusion such as memory lapses
- Irritated skin
- Puffy eyes

How to detox

The first step is to lighten your toxic load by eliminating all processed foods (refined and artificial and sugars, refined and bleached flours, hydrogenated and trans fats, gluten, chemicals in food and genetically modified foods), cigarettes, alcohol and coffee, all of which are received as toxins by your body and are an obstacle to the normal functioning of your body.

You should also minimize or better yet, eliminate the use of chemical-based detergents, household products, deodorant, and skin care products; and substitute them with organic and all natural alternatives.

Stress is another deterrent to good health as it triggers the release of stress hormones in your system. In large amounts these stress hormones override your detoxification enzymes in your liver. Meditation and yoga are some of the methods to help you deal with stress the right way.

The best ways to help your body detoxify

1. Drink at least eight glasses of water a day.
2. Eat plenty of negative calorie foods that are high fiber and that are organically grown. Radish, beets and edible seaweed are detoxifying super foods.
3. Take vitamin C rich foods. Vitamin C helps your body produce glutathione, a liver compound that eliminates toxins.
4. Cleanse and protect your liver by taking herbs such as milk thistle, dandelion root and burdock.
5. Practice swimmers breathing (deep breathing) to allow oxygen to circulate more effectively and completely through your system.
6. Go to a sauna to allow your body to eliminate toxins through perspiration.
7. Occasionally practice hydrotherapy by taking an extremely hot shower (as hot as you can handle) for five minutes; allowing the water to run down your body, especially your back. Follow this with very cold water for 30 seconds. Repeat this 3 times then take a nap for 30 minutes.
8. Dry brush your skin to drive toxins through your pores – look for special brushes in natural products department stores.

9. Exercising is a great way to detoxify. Fast jump roping and yoga are very effective. 30 minutes every day is enough time for an effective workout.

All day fat-flushing tea

1. Combine 8 cups of brewed green tea (unsweetened) with slices of lime, lemon and orange in a large pitcher.
2. Serve over ice or take it hot. You can refrigerate for up to 3 days.
3. Take 1 pitcher of this fat flushing tea a day for 5 days.

Give natural cleansing and detoxification an honest try and you are going to love how the Insulin resistance Diet is going to work for you in your weight loss journey and also in helping you transition to healthier long term eating habits.

We are now going to jump to the fun part of the book – meal plans.

We are doing all the work for you by sharing with you a 1 FULL Month meal plan that features some of the healthiest and tastiest recipes you've ever tasted. But first, get your apron ready and let's get cooking!

Chapter 13: Breakfast Recipes

Spicy Deviled Eggs

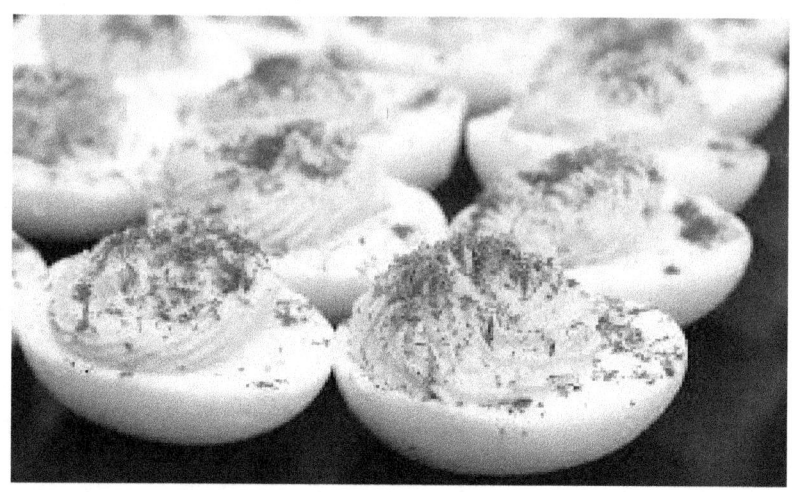

Prep time: 9 minutes

Cook time: 11 minutes

Serves: 2

Ingredients

- 4 hard-boiled eggs

- 2 tablespoon mayonnaise

- 1 tablespoon spicy brown mustard

- 1 tablespoon diced green chilies

Directions

1. Boil the eggs for 9 minutes.

2. Slice the eggs in half.

3. Scoop out the yolks.

4. Mix the yolks, the mayo, the mustard and the chilies.

5. Place back in the center of the egg whites.

6. Boil the eggs in advance and place in the fridge.

Nutritional Value: Calories: 202, Total Fat: 15g, Protein: 12g, Total Carbs: 3, Dietary Fiber: 0g, Sugar: 2g, Sodium: 20mg

Ham Rollups

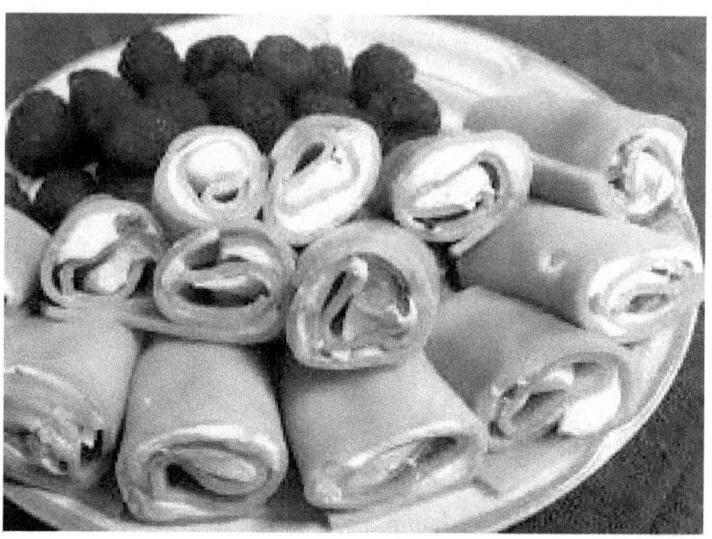

Prep time: 9 minutes

Cook time: 0 minutes

Serves: 6

Ingredients

- 6 Tortilla Factory low carb whole wheat tortillas

- 8 oz. whipped cream cheese

- 6 slices ham, the rectangular kind, cut in half

- ½ cup pickle dill relish

- 2 tablespoon mayonnaise

- 2 tablespoon Dijon mustard

Directions

1. Combine cream cheese, dill relish, mustard and mayo in a bowl.

2. Lay one tortilla out on waxed paper or saran wrap.

3. Place one slice of ham on top.

4. Spread ham slices with the cream cheese mixture.

5. Roll the entire piece up.

6. Cut in half.

7. Refrigerate until serving, 1 whole tortilla is one serving, so if cut in half, is still one serving.

8. Place serving size per individual zip-lock bag.

Nutritional Value: Calories: 228, Total Fat: 18g, Protein: 18g, Total Carbs: 6g, Dietary Fiber: 7g, Sugar: 0g, Sodium: 358mg

Butter Pecan Waffles

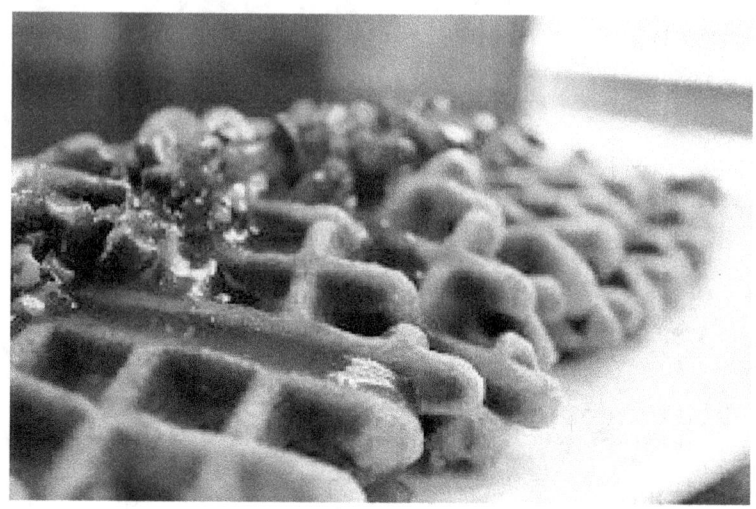

Prep time: 9 minutes

Cook time: 4 minutes

Serves: 8

Ingredients

- 1 cup soy flour

- 2 packets Splenda

- 3 tablespoon baking powder

- ¾ cup buttermilk

- 1 tablespoon butter

- ½ tablespoon baking soda

- 3 eggs

- 2 tablespoon vanilla

- ½ cup water

- 2 tablespoon sugar free butter rum flavoring

- ½ cup pecans

Directions

1. Combine everything except the pecans.

2. Use ¼ c batter for cooking the waffle.

3. Cook until crisp.

4. Top with pecans and sugar free syrup.

5. After the waffle is cool, place 1 per zip-lock bag. Warm by toasting in the toaster.

Nutritional Value: Calories: 181, Total Fat: 13g, Protein: 9g, Total Carbs: 5g, Dietary Fiber: 2g, Sugar: 3g, Sodium: 178mg

Breakfast Mexican Omelet

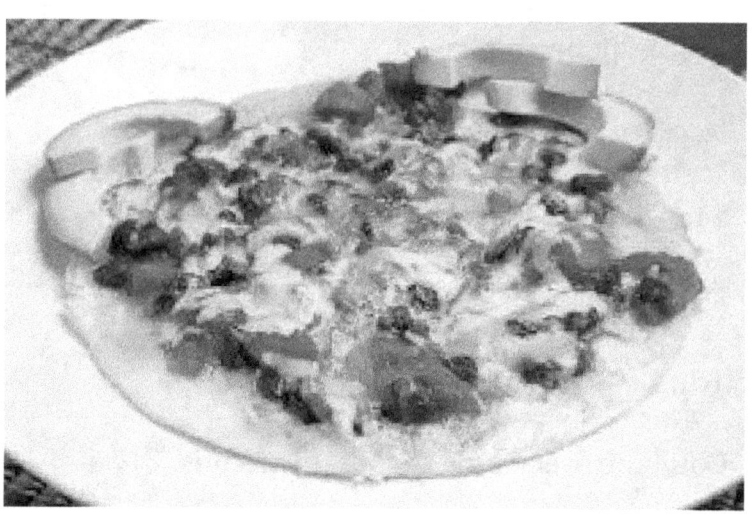

Prep time: 4 minutes

Cook time: 9 minutes

Serves: 1

Ingredients

- ½ tablespoon lime juice

- 2 eggs 1 tablespoon water

- 1 tablespoon crumbled bacon

- 1/2 tablespoon butter

- ¼ avocado

- ½ cup hand-shredded Mexican cheese

- 2 tablespoon Pace Thick and Chunky Medium Salsa

Directions

1. Melt the butter in a microwaveable bowl in the microwave.

2. Quickly whip the wet ingredients in a microwaveable bowl, can be the same bowl as before.

3. Microwave for one minute.

4. Place on warm plate.

5. Top with all the rest of the ingredients.

6. Combine the wet ingredients in a zip-lock bag, except the butter and water. Refrigerate. Combine the water and butter in a zip-lock bag.

Nutritional Value: Calories: 275, Total Fat: 21, Protein: 17g, Total Carbs: 3.2g, Dietary Fiber: 2g, Sugar: 2g, Sodium: 230mg

Cinnamon Chocolate Smoothie

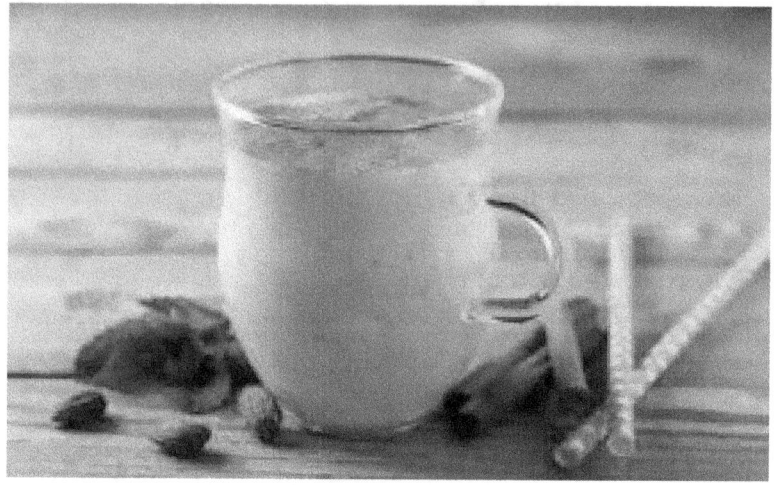

Prep time: 4 minutes

Cook time: 0 minutes

Serves: 1

Ingredients

- ½ cup firm Tofu

- 2 tablespoon cocoa powder

- 1 scoop chocolate protein powder

- 2 tablespoon cinnamon

- 2 sweetener packets

- 1 cup almond milk, unsweetened

- 4 ice cubes

Directions

1. Place all the ingredients in a blender, pulse until desired consistency, and serve.

2. Refrigerate the tofu. Place all the dry ingredients into one snack sized zip-lock bag.

Nutritional Value: Calories: 273, Total Fat: 15g, Protein: 33g, Total Carbs: 9g, Dietary Fiber: 20g, Sugar: 2g, Sodium: 214mg

Chocolate Muffin

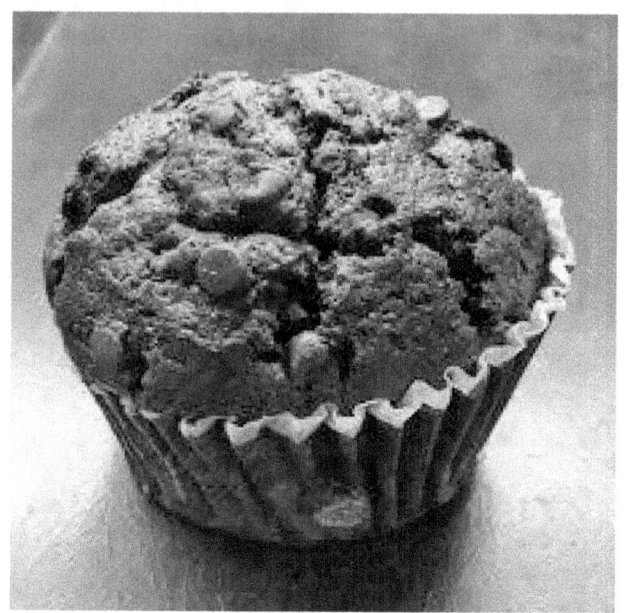

Prep time: 4 minutes

Cook time: 1 minutes

Serves: 1

Ingredients

- 1 tablespoon plain flour

- 1 scoop of Chocolate Protein Powder

- ½ tablespoon baking powder

- 1 tablespoon of cocoa powder

- 2 packets Splenda

- 1 tablespoon butter

- 1 egg

Directions

1. Mix the dry ingredients in a cup

2. Combine the wet ingredients

3. Add the wet ingredients into the cup of dry

4. Microwave for one minute

5. Place individual muffins in a zip-lock bag and place in the freezer. Microwave one minute to thaw and serve.

Nutritional Value: Calories: 207, Total Fat: 24g, Protein: 10g, Total Carbs: 16, Dietary Fiber: 11g, Sugar: 0, Sodium: 308mg

Denver Omelet

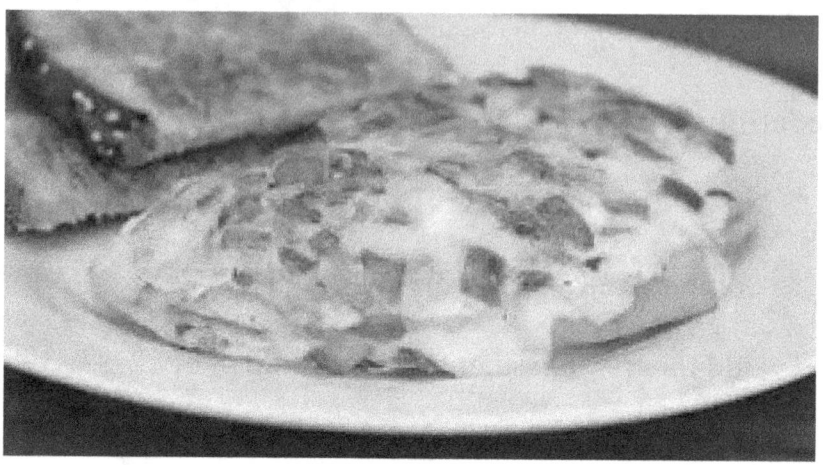

Prep time: 4 minutes

Cook time: 1 minutes

Serves: 1

Ingredients

- 2 tablespoon butter

- ¼ cup chopped onions

- ¼ cup green bell pepper, diced

- ¼ cup halved grape tomatoes

- 2 eggs

- ¼ cup chopped ham

Directions

1. Sautee the onions and bell pepper, with the butter, in a small skillet.

2. Whip the eggs and mix the ingredients in a bowl.

3. Microwave for one minute.

4. Pre-cook the peppers and onions and place in zip-lock freezer bags by portions, add the ham to the bags. Freeze. The night before making, place the peppers mix in the fridge to thaw or microwave for one minute before adding to the whipped egg to make.

Nutritional Value: Calories: 605, Total Fat: 46g, Protein: 39g, Total Carbs: 6g, Dietary Fiber: 2g, Sugar: 0g, Sodium: 380mg

Cheese Blintz with Blueberries

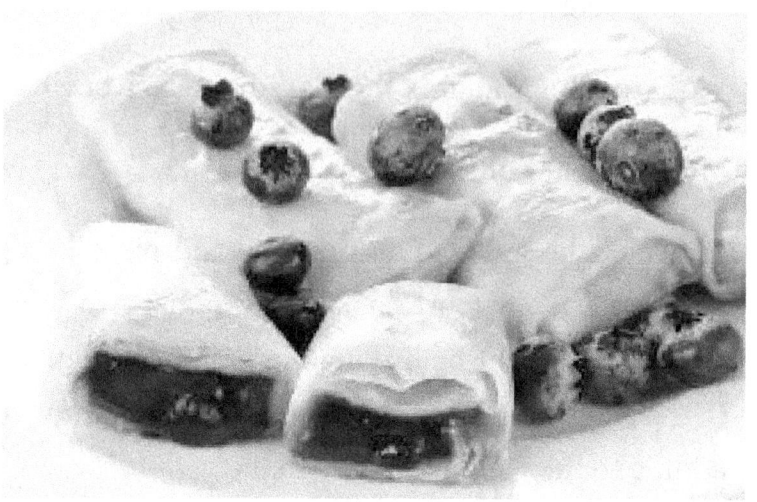

Prep time: 9 minutes

Cook time: 4 minutes

Serves: 1

Ingredients

- 1 medium egg

- 1 tablespoon half & half

- 1 scoop protein shake powder, vanilla

- 1 pat of butter

- 1 tablespoon of olive oil

- 2 tablespoon ricotta cheese

- 1 tablespoon Greek yogurt, plain

- 1 packet sweetener

- 1 tablespoon cinnamon

- ½ cup blueberries

Directions

1. Combine the ricotta cheese, Greek yogurt, sweetener and cinnamon in a bowl, mix well.

2. Combine the egg, protein powder, and cream. Whisk until all lumps are dissolved, and the mixture is well-blended.

3. Coat a non-stick skillet with the olive oil.

4. At medium heat, melt butter in the skillet and pour the batter on top.

5. Swirl the skillet until the batter is evenly distributed. When the batter has set, gently turn the blintz to the other side.

6. Let cook for one minute until the batter is set, but not browned.

7. Gently fold half the blueberries into the filling.

8. Place the filling in the middle of the blitz.

9. Roll into a pancake and serve with the remaining blueberries.

10. Mix the filling and place in the fridge in a covered container. Place the blueberries in a zip-lock bag and place in the freezer.

Nutritional Value: Calories: 427 Total Fat: 23g, Protein: 39g, Total Carbs: 14g, Dietary Fiber: 3g, Sugar: 10g, Sodium: 330mg

Huevos Rancheros

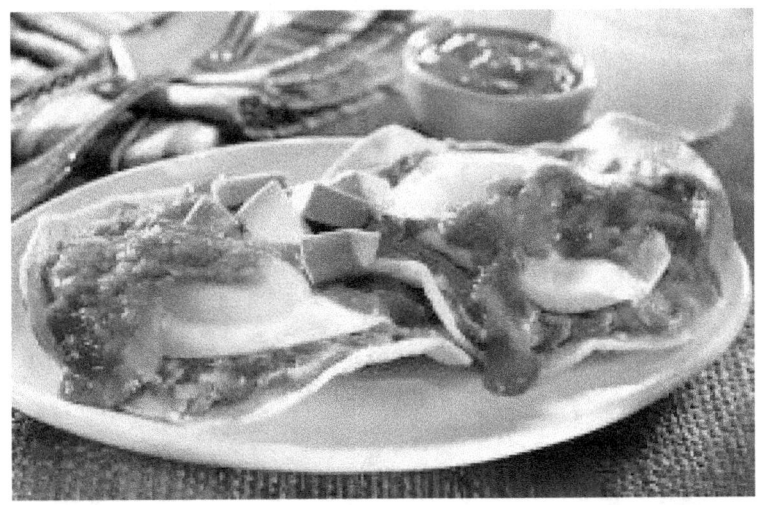

Prep time: 9 minutes

Cook time: 19 minutes

Serves: 4

Ingredients

- 4 oz. cooked ground sirloin

- ½ cup Pace Salsa Verde

- 4 eggs

- 4 slices Canadian bacon

- 4 Tortilla Factory Low Carb Whole Wheat tortillas

- 4 tablespoon water

- 4 tablespoon butter

Directions

1. Melt the butter in a glass bowl.

2. Quickly whip the egg and water with the butter.

3. Microwave 1 minute.

4. Place the tortilla in the microwave for 10 seconds.

5. Layer as follows: Tortilla, Canadian bacon, ground beef, egg, salsa.

6. Place Canadian bacon, cooked sirloin, and salsa into a zip-lock bag. Freeze or refrigerate. Place the tortillas in the fridge to keep them fresh. Add the eggs, etc. when microwaving

Nutritional Value: Calories: 277, Total Fat: 17g, Protein: 20g, Total Carbs: 8g, Dietary Fiber: 13g, Sugar: 3g, Sodium: 720mg

Sausage Egg Muffins

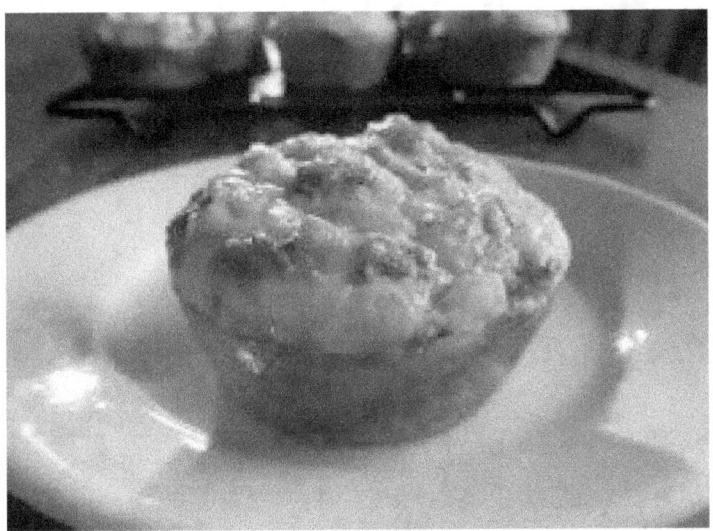

Prep time: 10minutes

Cook time: 29 minutes

Serves: 12

Ingredients

- 12 oz. cooked sausage crumbles

- 12 eggs

- ¼ cup milk

- 2 cups cheddar cheese, sharp, hand-shredded

- ¼ tablespoon black pepper or chili pepper

Directions

1. Mix all the ingredients.

2. Pour into 12 greased muffin papers (in a pan).

3. Bake at 375 degrees for 29 minutes.

4. Cool for 4 minutes before serving.

Freezing Instructions

5. After cooling, place in zip-lock freezer bag. For the best flavor, heat in microwave or toaster oven before eating.

Nutritional Value: Calories: 200, Total Fat: 39g, Protein: 16g, Total Carbs: 2g, Dietary Fiber: 0g, Sugar: 0, Sodium: 370mg

Junior Mint Shake

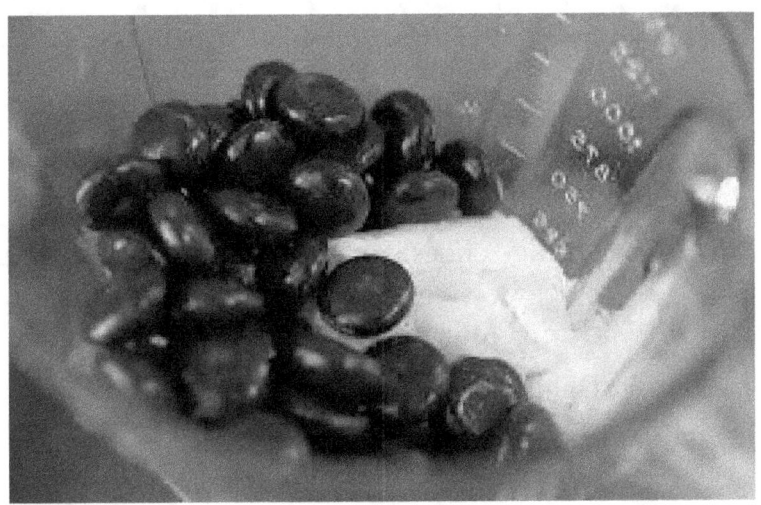

Prep time: 4 minutes

Cook time: 0

Serves: 1

Ingredients

- 2 tablespoon cocoa

- 6 oz. COLD water

- ¼ cup protein powder or chocolate

- 3 drops peppermint flavoring

- ½ cup cottage cheese

- 2 packets sweetener

- 5 ice cubes

Directions

1. Mix the ingredients and emulsify by blending.

2. Blend until thick.

3. Combine dry ingredients and place in zip-lock bag. Combine cottage cheese and sweetener and refrigerate.

Nutritional Value: Calories: 200, Total Fat: 2g, Protein: 39g, Total Carbs: 7g, Dietary Fiber: 1g, Sugar: 3g, Sodium: 348mg

Spinach and Swiss Quiche

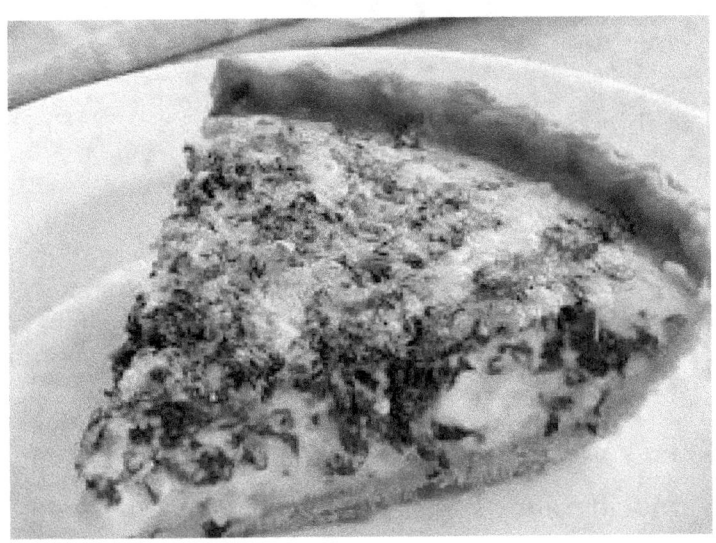

Prep time: 19 minutes

Cook time: 29 minutes

Serves: 4

Ingredients

- 2 tablespoon butter

- 6 oz. frozen chopped spinach, drained and thawed

- 1 cup cream

- 1 cup hand-shredded swiss cheese or hand-shredded cheese

- ¼ tablespoon salt

- 1 diced white onion

- 4 eggs

- ⅛ tablespoon nutmeg

- ¼ tablespoon black pepper, ground

Directions

1. Heat the oven to 350 degrees.

2. Then spray a pie pan with your choice of cooking spray. Spray liberally as eggs may stick.

3. Cook onions in butter till glassy, then add the spinach and simmer until the water is gone.

4. Mix all of the ingredients in a bowl, including the spices.

5. Pour into the pie pan.

6. Bake for 29 minutes.

7. Cool for 9 minutes and cut into quarters.

8. Wrap a cooled slice of quiche in saran wrap, then place in a zip-lock bag. Microwave for 1 minute in two 30-second bursts.

Nutritional Value: Calories: 417, Total Fat: 37g, Protein: 15g, Total Carbs: 4g, Dietary Fiber: 1.5g, Sugar: 0g, Sodium: 209mg

Chapter 14: Lunch

Chili Mac

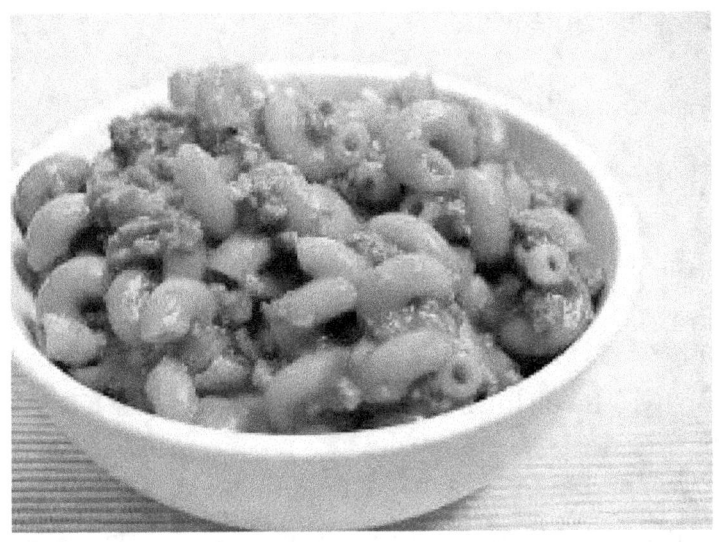

Prep time: 9 minutes

Cook time: 9 minutes

Serves: 4

Ingredients

- 1 lb ground Sirloin

- 1 chopped Onion

- 1 Chili Seasoning Mix, packet

- 1 cup tomato sauce

- 1 small can of Chunky Diced Tomatoes & Green Chilies

- 1 cup hand-shredded sharp cheddar

- 1 packet Splenda

- ½ cup Barilla Proteinplus Elbow macaroni

Directions

1. Boil Barilla Proteinplus Elbow macaroni until done, drain.

2. Brown the sirloin and onions in a large skillet.

3. Add the pasta, tomato sauce, diced tomatoes and green chilies, and chili seasoning mix.

4. Taste to see if you need to add water.

5. Serve in 4 bowls, topping each bowl with the cheddar cheese.

6. Place in four containers with lids, freeze. Microwave 2 minutes to thaw.

Nutritional Value: Calories: 480, Total Fat: 24g, Protein: 36g, Total Carbs: g, 25Dietary Fiber: 6g, Sugar: 4g, Sodium: 995mg

Cobb Salad

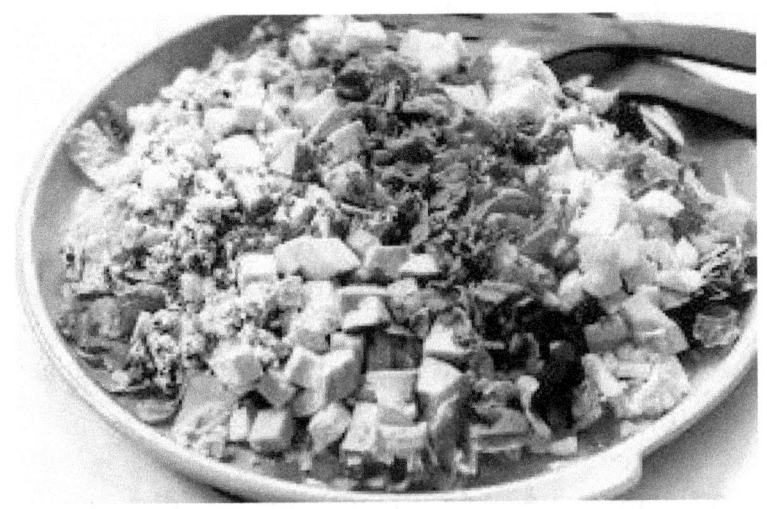

Prep time: 9 minutes

Cook time: 9 minutes

Serves: 1

Ingredients

- 1 slice Bacon or 1 tablespoon real bacon bits

- 1 grilled Chicken Breast, which has been cut into thin strips

- 1 cup Spring Mix Salad

- 1/2 cup grape tomatoes, sliced in half

- ½ avocado, sliced into small moons

- ¼ cup pepper jack cheese, hand-shredded

- 2 tablespoon Ken's Buttermilk Ranch Dressing

Directions

1. Assemble ingredients by sections.

2. Cover the entire bottom of the plate with lettuce.

3. In one corner (relative if you have a round plate) place the tomatoes.

4. In the opposite section place the avocado strips in a fan shape.

5. In the third section place the bacon bits.

6. In the fourth section place the hand-shredded cheese. In the center place the chicken.

7. Drizzle with the salad dressing and serve.

8. The chicken can be frozen in a zip-lock bag. Microwave 1 minute to serve. The salad can be combined in one bowl or packed in individual containers and placed in the fridge.

Nutritional Value: Calories: 561, Total Fat: 34g, Protein: 51g, Total Carbs: 3.9g, Dietary Fiber: 6g, Sugar: 1g, Sodium: 802mg

Stuffed with goat cheese,

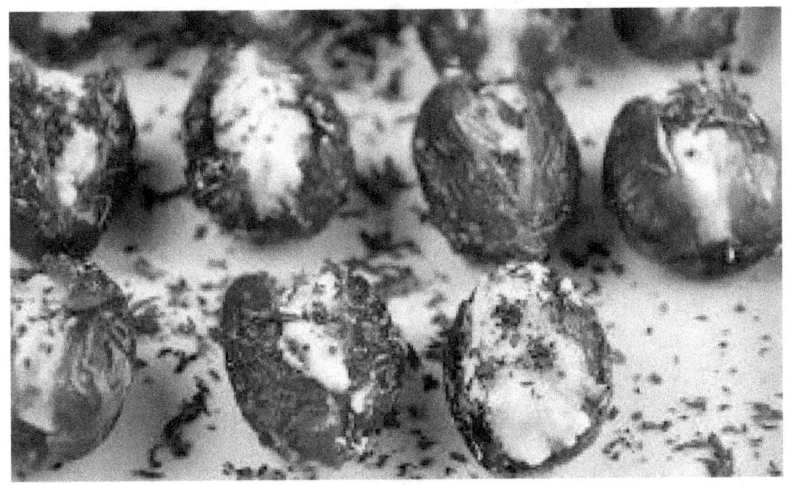

Prep Time: 5 Hours and 30 Minutes

Serves: 4

Ingredients:

- ¼ cup of red wine

- ¼ cup of balsamic vinegar

- 2 tablespoon of Dijon mustard

- 2 tablespoon of soy sauce

- 1 cup of extra virgin olive oil

- 4 cloves of garlic, peeled and thinly sliced

- 1 tablespoon of salt Dash of black pepper

- 1, 2 to 3 pounds of flank steak

Ingredients for the stuffing:

- ½ cup of pancetta, cooked and chopped

- 8 ounces of goat cheese

- 3 cups of spinach, drained and excess liquid drained

Directions:

1. Use a large bowl and add in the red wine, vinegar, mustard, soy sauce, olive oil, garlic and dash of salt and black pepper. Whisk until mixed.

2. Add in the flank steak and cover. Set in the fridge to marinate for 4 hours.

3. Place a large saucepan over low heat. Chop the pancetta and place into the saucepan. Cook for 20 to 30 minutes. Drain the excess fat and set the pancetta aside.

4. Add the spinach into the saucepan and cook for 1 to 2 minutes or until fragrant. Remove from the pan and squeeze out the excess liquid. Add into a bowl with the pancetta and goat cheese. Stir well to mix.

5. Remove the flank steak from the marinade and place onto a flat surface. Beat with a meat mallet until ¼ inch in thickness.

6. Spread the stuffing onto the flank steak. Roll and tie with twine to seal. Season with a dash of salt and black pepper.

7. Heat up the oven to 400 degrees.

8. Place the rolled flank steak onto a large baking sheet and drizzle a few drops of olive oil over the top.

9. Place into the oven to bake for 15 to 25 minutes or until cooked through. Remove and allow to rest for 15 minutes before serving.

Nutritional Value: Calories: 646, Fat: 58 grams, Carbs: 4 grams, Protein: 27 grams

Chicken Quesadillas

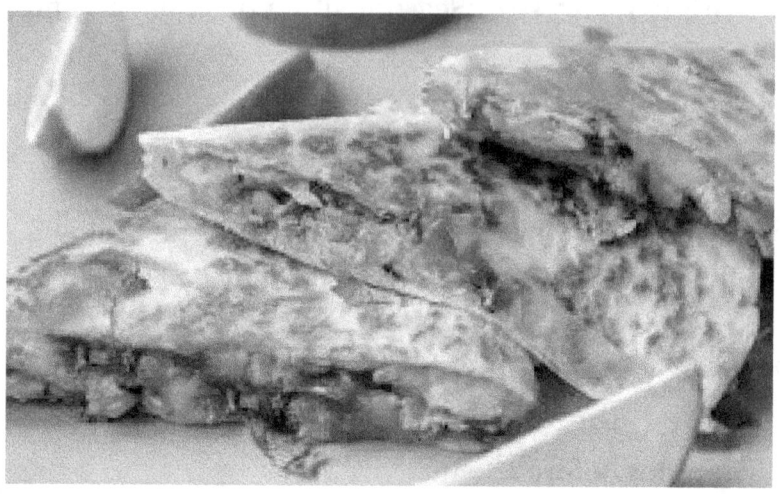

Prep time: 4 minutes

Cook time: 4 minutes

Serves: 4

Ingredients

- 1 cup pepper jack cheese, hand-shredded

- 8 tortillas Tortilla Factory Low Carb Whole Wheat Tortillas

- 8 oz. cooked and shredded Chicken Breast

- 1 chopped and Roasted Bell Pepper

- 2 tablespoon Cilantro

- 2 tablespoon Butter

- 1 cup plain Greek yogurt

Directions

1. Place ½ pat of butter in a skillet

2. Mix all the ingredients in a bowl except the yogurt

3. Place meat ingredients inside tortillas

4. Toast each side

5. Cut into 4 wedges

6. Top with yogurt and salsa, if desired

7. Freeze in zip-lock bags. Place the yogurt in the fridge. Heat one minute in the microwave to thaw.

Nutritional Value: Calories: 425g, Total Fat: 25g, Protein: 44g, Total Carbs: 10g, Dietary Fiber: 9g, Sugar: 2g, Sodium: 186mg

Chicken Lettuce Wraps

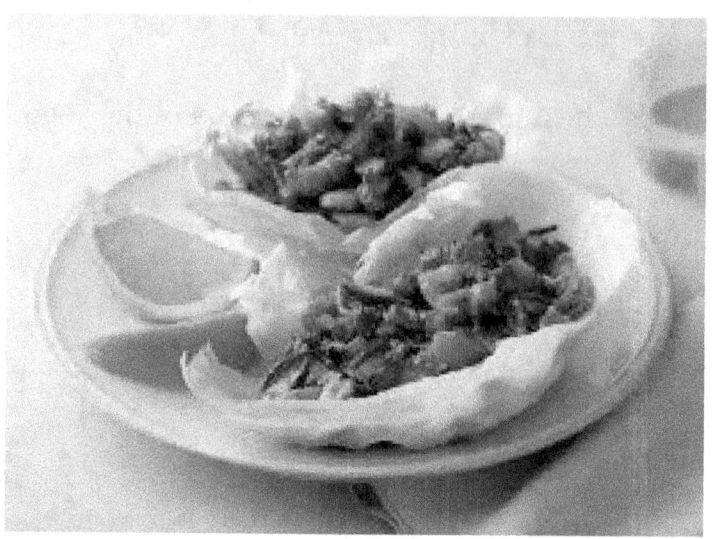

Prep time: 10minutes

Cook time: 10minutes

Serves: 1

Ingredients

- 1 chicken breast, boneless, diced into 1-inch size pieces

- 1 cup diced or sliced fresh mushrooms

- ½ cup diced water chestnuts (from a can, drained)

- 1 tablespoon olive oil

- 1 tablespoon onion, minced

- 1 tablespoon minced garlic

- 1 tablespoon teriyaki sauce

- garlic powder, only a dash

- onion powder, just a dash

- oregano, one dash

- cayenne pepper, a small dash

- salt /pepper

Directions

1. Mix the ingredients and cook in a skillet until the chicken is done, about 10 minutes.

2. Shred the chicken

3. Place in leaves and roll

4. Place all ingredients into one freezer bag except the lettuce. Microwave one minute and serve.

Nutritional Value: Calories: 145, Total Fat: 1g, Protein: 35g, Dietary Fiber: 1g, Total Carbs: 4g, Sugar: 0g, Sodium: 100mg

Seven Layer Salad

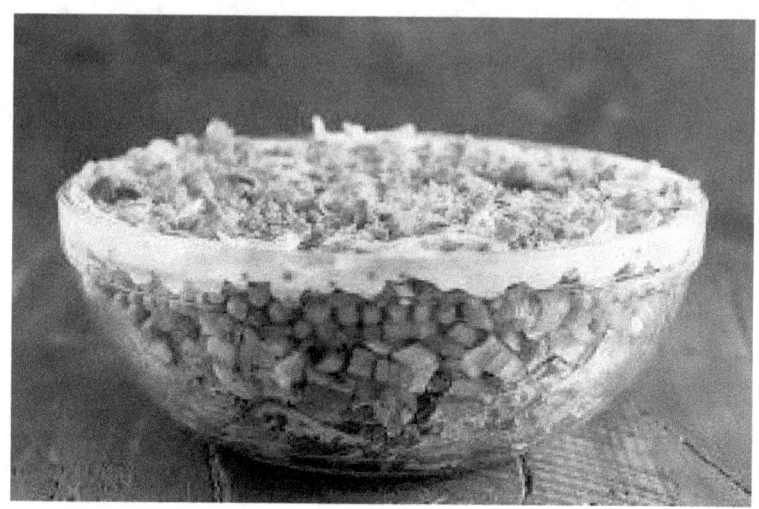

Prep time: 14 minutes

Cook time: 9 minutes

Serves: 10

Ingredients

- 4 cups shredded butter lettuce
- 4 cups shredded romaine lettuce
- 1 cup peas
- 1 cup diced bell peppers, red and yellow
- 1 cup grape tomatoes, halved
- 1 cup sliced celery
- ½ cup red onion
- ¾ cup Greek yogurt
- ¾ cup mayonnaise

- 2 tablespoon garlic powder

- 1 tablespoon dill

- 2 tablespoon lemon juice

- 2 English cucumbers, chopped with peels on

- 2 tablespoon olive oil

- ¼ tablespoon black pepper

- 1 small can black olives, sliced and drained (2.25 oz. can)

- ½ tablespoon mint or 3 mint leaves

Directions

1. Combine Greek yogurt, dill, garlic powder, mint, lemon juice, olive oil, ½ cup diced cucumber, and black pepper and emulsify by blending.

2. Taste and add salt. Add water by tablespoons if too thick.

3. Arrange on 4 plates the lettuce and spinach, tomatoes, cucumbers, and black olives.

4. Pour the dressing over the salad.

5. Top with the feta cheese.

6. Mix the salad dressing and place in fridge in closed containers. Mix the salad and bag or place in covered containers in the fridge.

7. Place the feta cheese in a zip-lock bag in the fridge.

Nutritional Value: Calories: 142, Total Fat: 10g, Protein: 4g, Total Carbs: 7g, Dietary Fiber: 3g, Sugar: 0g, Sodium: 144mg

Shrimp and Cucumber Salad

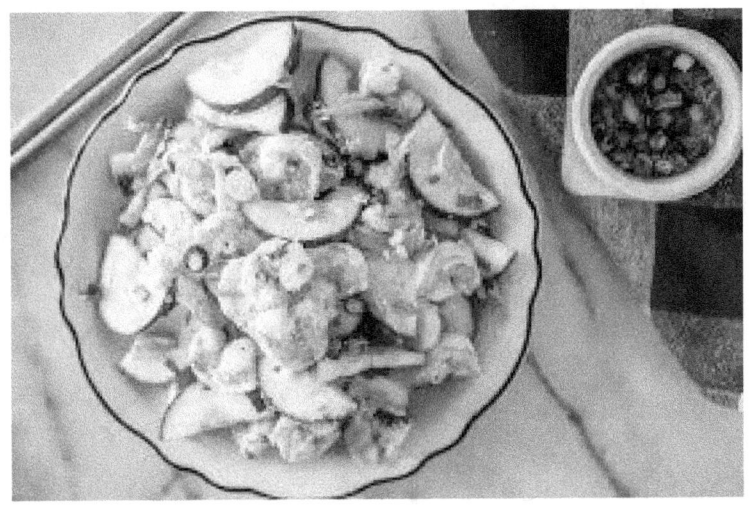

Prep time: 4 minutes

Cook time: 0 minutes

Serves: 4

Ingredients

- 2 English cucumbers

- 1/4 cup of red wine vinegar

- 2 tablespoon of Splenda

- 1/4 tablespoon salt

- ½ cup cooked shrimp

Directions

1. Peel the cucumbers so that they have stripes down the side.

2. Slice the cucumbers as thin as you can.

3. Mix the dressing of sugar, salt, and vinegar very well

4. Place the cucumbers on a plate

5. Place the shrimp on top

6. Add the dressing and serve.

7. Create the entire salad and place in a covered container in the fridge. Will keep 2 days.

Nutritional Value: Calories: 26g, Total Fat: 0g, Protein: 2g, Total Carbs: 3g, Dietary Fiber: 2g, Sugar: 2g, Sodium: 157mg

Chapter 16: Dinner

Italian Meatballs

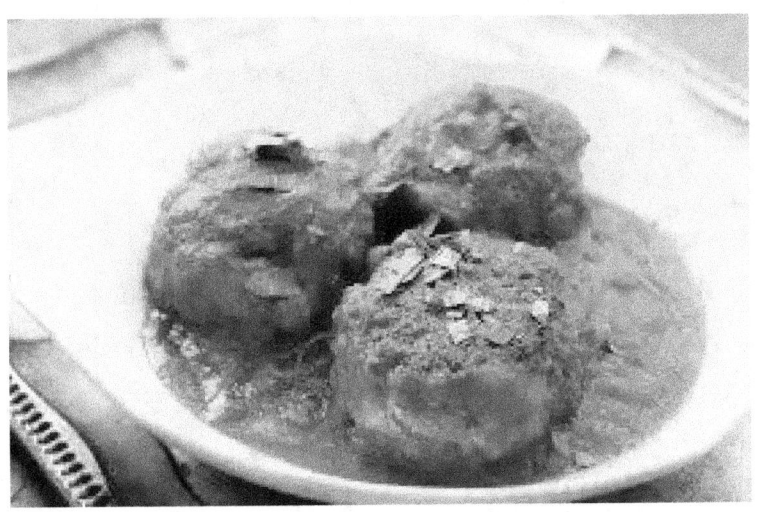

Prep Time: 40 Minutes

Serves: 4

Ingredients:

- 1 pound of beef, lean and ground

- 1 tablespoon of Italian seasoning

- 1 tablespoon of garlic, granulated

- ½ tablespoon of onion, powdered

- 2 tablespoon of salt

- ½ tablespoon of black pepper

- 1 tablespoon of Worcestershire sauce

- 2 tablespoon of tomato paste

- 1 egg, large

- 2 tablespoon of flaxseed meal

- ¼ cup of Parmesan cheese, grated

- ¼ cup of mozzarella cheese, shredded

Directions:

1. Use a large bowl and add in the ground beef, Italian seasoning, garlic, onion, a dash of salt and black pepper, Worcestershire sauce and tomato paste. Stir well to mix.

2. Add the remaining ingredients into the bowl and stir well to mix.

3. Preheat the oven to 400 degrees.

4. While the oven is heating up, form the mixture into even sized meatballs. Place the meatballs onto a lightly greased baking sheet.

5. Place into the oven to bake for 20 minutes or until cooked through.

6. Remove and serve immediately with a meal of your choice.

Nutritional Value: Calories: 451, Fat: 39 grams, Carbs: 3 grams, Protein: 22 grams

Healthy Kale Chicken Caesar Salad

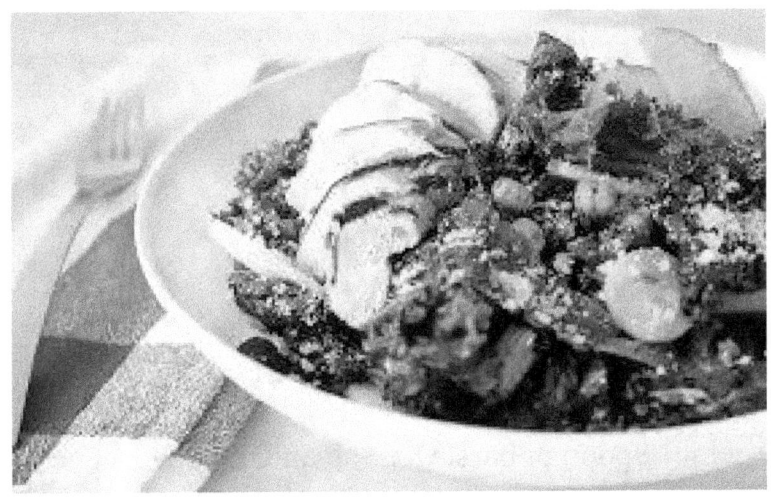

Prep Time: 35 Minutes

Serves: 8

Ingredients for the salad:

- 2 chicken breasts, boneless and skinless

- 4 tablespoon of extra virgin olive oil

- 2 tablespoon of salt

- ½ tablespoon of black pepper

- 1 tablespoon of garlic, powdered

- 1 bunch of kale, washed, chopped and with ribs removed

Ingredients for the salad dressing:

- 1 egg yolk, large

- 2 anchovies

- 1 lemon, fresh and juice only

- 1 tablespoon of apple cider

- ¼ cup of parmesan cheese, grated

- 2 tablespoon of parsley, fresh and chopped

- Dash of salt and black pepper

- ¼ cup of extra virgin olive oil

- 1 to 2 tablespoon of water

Directions:

1. First, preheat the oven to 375 degrees.

2. While the oven is heating up add the chicken breasts into a large bowl. Add in the extra virgin olive oil, dash of salt and black pepper and garlic. Toss well to mix.

3. Place the chicken breasts onto a large baking sheet. Place into the oven to bake for 30 minutes. Remove after this time and slice the chicken into thin strips.

4. Use a food processor and add in all of the ingredients for the salad dressing except for the oil. Blend on the highest setting until smooth in consistency. Then slowly pour in the oil while blending until the dressing is emulsified.

5. Place the kale in a large serving bowl. Add in the chicken and salad dressing. Toss well to mix. Serve immediately.

Nutritional Value: Calories: 208, Fat: 16 grams, Carbs: 8 grams, Protein: 8 grams

Smothered Pan Seared Salmon

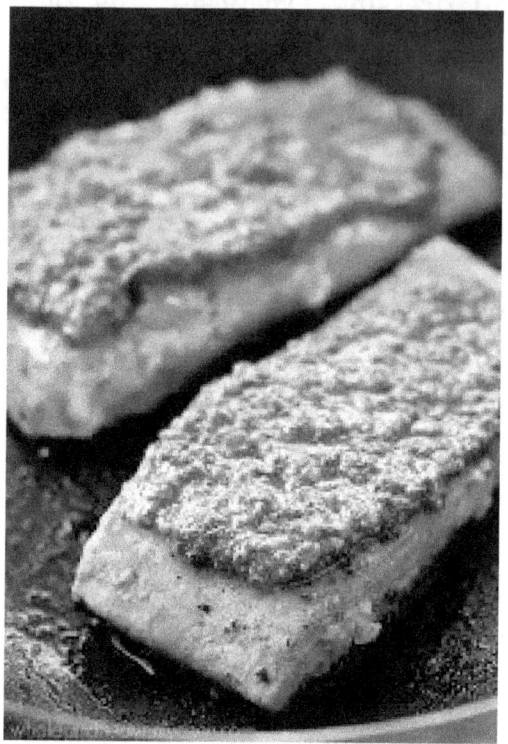

Prep Time: 20 Minutes

Serves: 4

Ingredients:

- 4, 4 ounce salmon fillets

- 2 tablespoon of coconut oil 1

- Tablespoon of salt

- ½ tablespoon of black pepper

- 1 tablespoon of garlic, powdered

- 1 tablespoon of onion, powdered

- 4 tablespoon of butter

- ½ cup of Greek yogurt, plain

- ½ cup of sour cream

- 2 tablespoon of extra virgin olive

- 1 tablespoon of dill, dried

- 1 lemon, fresh and juice only

- Dash of Tabasco sauce

Directions:

1. Use a medium bowl and add in the salt, black pepper, garlic, and onion. Stir well to mix. Sprinkle this mixture over the salmon fillets. Set the remaining seasoning aside.

2. Place a large skillet over medium to high heat. Add in the coconut oil and once the oil is hot enough add in the salmon fillets. Cook for 3 minutes on each side. Flip and continue to cook for another 3 minutes. Remove and set the salmon aside.

3. Add a tablespoon of butter over each salmon fillet.

4. Add the remaining seasoning, plain yogurt and sour cream into the skillet. Whisk until smooth in consistency. Cook for a further 2 to 3 minutes.

5. Remove from heat and pour the sauce over the top. Serve.

Nutritional Value: Calories: 558, Fat: 58 grams, Carbs: 3 grams, Protein: 24 grams

Oven Roasted Broccoli with Parmesan Cheese and Garlic

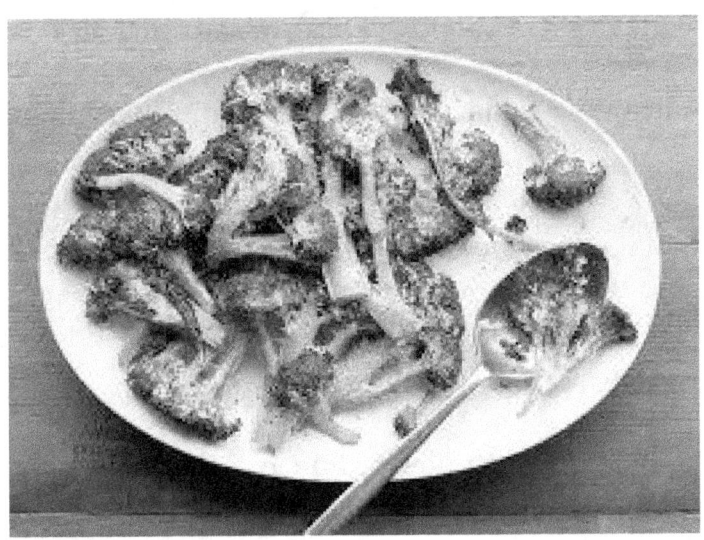

Prep Time: 20 Minutes

Serves: 4

Ingredients:

- 1 head of broccoli, fresh and cut into florets

- 2 cloves of garlic, minced

- ¼ cup of extra virgin olive oil

- Dash of salt and black pepper

- 8 tablespoon of parmesan cheese, grated and divided

- ½ of a lemon, fresh and juice only

Directions:

1. In a medium bowl add in the broccoli florets, garlic, extra virgin olive oil and dash of salt and black pepper.

2. Add in six tablespoons of the grated Parmesan cheese into the mixture and stir well to mix.

3. Add the seasoned broccoli onto a large baking sheet.

4. Place into the oven to roast at 400 degrees for 15 to 20 minutes.

5. Remove from the oven. Squeeze the fresh lemon juice over the top.

6. Sprinkle the remaining Parmesan cheese over the top and toss to coat. Serve.

Nutritional Value: Calories: 242, Fat: 18 grams, Carbs: 11 grams, Protein: 9 grams

Tilapia and Broccoli

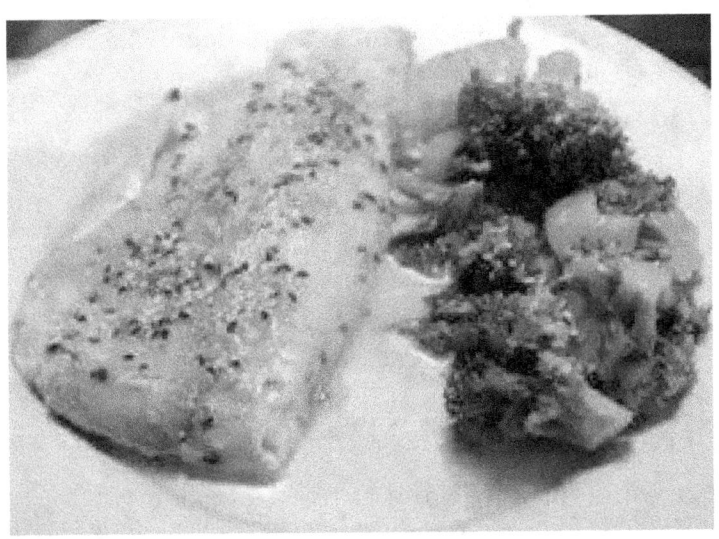

Prep time: 4 minutes

Cook time: 14 minutes

Serves: 1

Ingredients

- 6 oz. tilapia, frozen is fine

- 1 tablespoon butter

- 1 tablespoon garlic, minced or finely chopped

- 1 tablespoon of lemon pepper seasoning

- 1 cup broccoli florets, fresh or frozen, but fresh will be crisper

Directions

1. Set the pre-warmed oven for 350 degrees.

2. Place the fish in an aluminum foil packet.

3. Arrange the broccoli around the fish to make an attractive arrangement.

4. Sprinkle the lemon pepper on the fish.

5. Close the packet and seal, bake for 14 minutes.

6. Combine the garlic and butter. Set aside.

7. Remove the packet from the oven and transfer ingredients to a plate.

8. Place the butter on the fish and broccoli.

9. Place the butter and garlic into small sealed containers or zip-lock bags, Refrigerate or freeze. Cut the broccoli (if fresh) and place in zip-lock bags in the fridge. Place the lemon pepper into a small container.

Nutritional Value: Calories: 362, Total Fat: 25g, Protein: 29g, Total Carbs: 3.5g, Dietary Fiber: 3g, Sugar: 0g, Sodium: 0mg

Hangar Steak

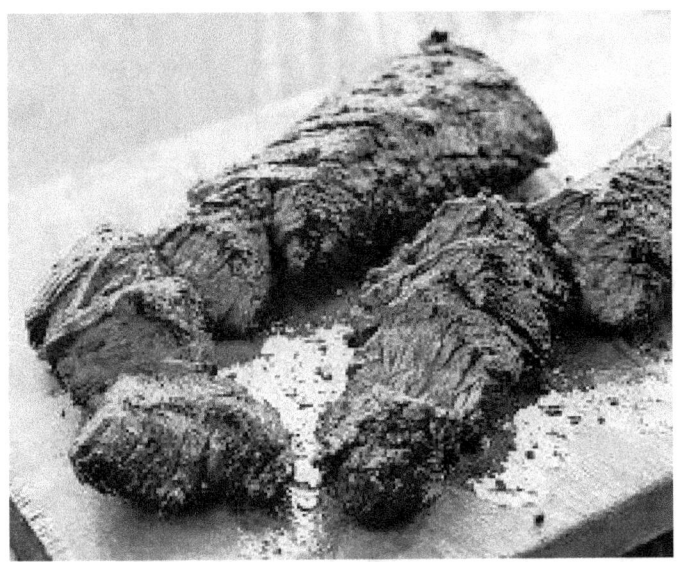

Prep Time: 4 Hours and 15 Minutes

Serves: 8

Ingredients:

- 2 pounds of hanger steak, cleaned and trimmed

- 1 tablespoon of salt

- 1 tablespoon of black pepper

- 1 tablespoon of garlic, granulated

- ½ cup of extra virgin olive

- 2 tablespoon of soy sauce

- 2 tablespoon of vinegar, red wine

- ½ cup of red wine

- 2 tablespoon of rosemary, fresh

- 1 stick of butter, melted

Directions:

1. Add all of the ingredients except for the hangar steak and melted butter into a large bowl. Stir well until evenly mixed.

2. Add in the hangar steak and toss to coat. Cover and set in the fridge to marinate for 4 hours.

3. After this time preheat an outdoor grill to medium heat.

4. Place the marinated steak onto the grill. Grill for 5 to 10 minutes on each side or until cooked to the desired doneness.

5. Remove from the grill and drizzle the melted butter over the steak. Serve.

Nutritional Value: Calories: 338, Fat: 26 grams, Carbs: 1 gram, Protein: 25 grams

Simple Salisbury Steak

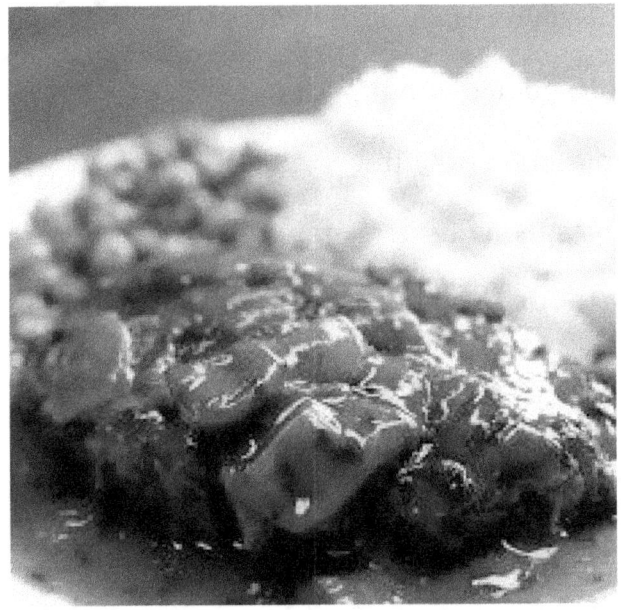

Prep Time: 20 Minutes

Serves: 8

Ingredients for the steak:

- 3 pounds of beef, lean and ground

- ½ cup of panko breadcrumbs

- 2 eggs, large

- 2 tablespoon of ketchup, low in sugar

- 4 tablespoon of mustard, dried

- 8 dashes of Worcestershire sauce

- 1 tablespoon of salt

- 1 tablespoon of black pepper

- 1 tablespoon of garlic, powdered

- 1 tablespoon of onion, powdered

- 2 tablespoon of butter

- 2 tablespoon of extra virgin olive oil

Ingredients for the gravy:

- 1 onion, sliced thinly

- 4 cups of beef broth

- 2 tablespoon of ketchup, low in sugar

- 2 tablespoon of kitchen bouquet

- 8 dashes of Worcestershire sauce

- 2 tablespoon of cornstarch

Directions:

1. Use a large bowl and add in all of the ingredients for the steak except for the butter and extra virgin olive oil. Stir well to mix and form this mixture into patties.

2. Place a large saucepan over medium heat. Add in the extra virgin olive oil and butter. As soon as the butter melts add in the beef patties. Cook for 8 minutes on each side or until cooked through.

3. Remove the cooked patties from the skillet and transfer to a large plate.

4. Add the sliced onions into the skillet. Cook for 5 to 10 minutes or until soft.

5. Then add in the beef broth, low sugar ketchup, kitchen bouquet and Worcestershire sauce. Whisk until smooth in consistency.

6. Add in the cornstarch and whisk to mix. Continue to cook for an additional 2 minutes or until thick in consistency.

7. Add the cooked patties into the gravy and toss to mix.

8. Remove from heat and serve.

Nutritional Value: Calories: 519, Fat: 59 grams, Carbs: 18 grams, Protein: 29 grams

Classic Prime Rib

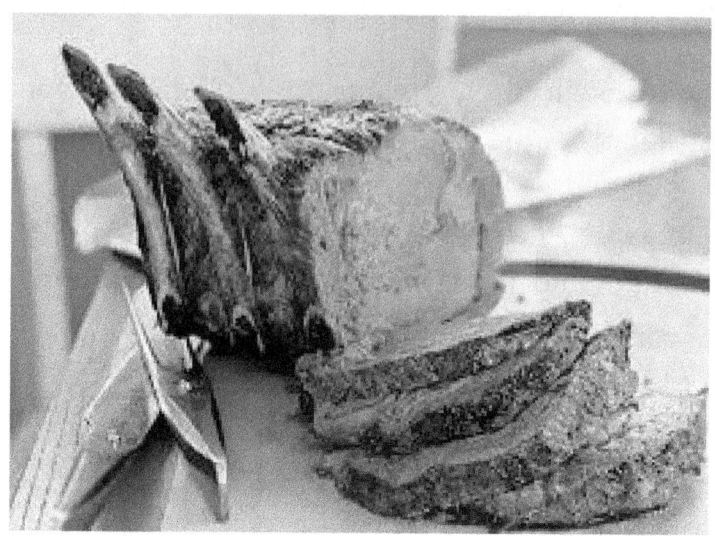

Prep Time: 3 Hours

Serves: 3

Ingredients for the prime rib:

- 1, 8 to 12 pound prime rib, boneless
- ¼ cup of extra virgin olive oil
- ½ cup of salt
- 1 tablespoon of black pepper
- 2 tablespoon of garlic, granulated
- 1 tablespoon of thyme, dried
- 1 tablespoon of rosemary, dried
- 2 tablespoon of smoked paprika

Ingredients for the horseradish cream:

- 1 cup of sour cream

- ½ cup of mayonnaise
- ¼ cup of horseradish, drained
- ½ of a lemon, juice
- Dash of Tabasco sauce
- Dash of salt and black pepper

Directions:

1. Score the skin of the prime rib with a knife.

2. Drizzle the olive oil over the prime rib. Season with: garlic, thyme, rosemary, paprika and dash of salt and black pepper.

3. Then preheat the oven to 450 to 500 degrees.

4. Place the seasoned prime rib onto a large baking sheet. Place into the oven to roast for 20 minutes. After this time increase the oven to broil and broil for another 8 minutes. Reduce the temperature of the oven to 325 degrees. Roast for 1 hour and 20 minutes.

5. Remove from the oven and set aside to rest for 30 minutes. Slice and serve.

Nutritional Value: Calories: 640, Fat: 56 grams, Carbs: 2 grams, Protein: 33 grams

Zucchini Casserole

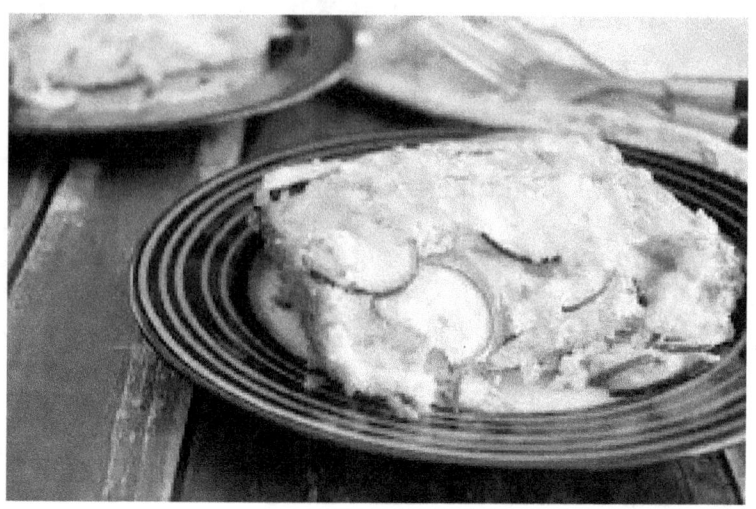

Prep Time: 1 Hour

Serves: 8

Ingredients:

- 5 pieces of bacon, chopped

- 1 onion, chopped

- 2 cloves of garlic, minced

- 2 cups of zucchini, grated

- 1 cup of Colby Jack cheese, grated

- ½ cup of almond flour

- ½ cup of vegetable oil

- ¼ cup of heavy cream

- 6 eggs, large

- Dash of salt and black pepper

Directions:

1. Place a large skillet over low to medium heat. Add in the bacon and cook for 5 minutes or until browned. Transfer the bacon to a large plate lined with paper towels to drain.

2. In the skillet with the bacon fat. Add in the onion and garlic. Stir well to mix and cook for 5 minutes or until soft. Transfer the mixture into a large bowl.

3. Add in the remaining ingredients into the bowl. Whisk well to mix and pour into a large greased baking dish.

4. Top the casserole with the shredded Colby Jack cheese.

5. Place into the oven to bake for 1 hour at 350 degrees. Make sure to turn the casserole after 30 minutes of baking.

6. Remove and allow to cool for 5 minutes before serving.

Nutritional Value: Calories: 334, Fat: 30 grams, Carbs: 6 grams, Protein: 12 grams

In Conclusion

I hope this book was able to help you to find your way through the potentially fearful terrain of waking up to, temporarily living with, and moving past a state of insulin resistance.

With the steps outlined in this book as a guide, you won't become another statistic. You will join the pioneering ranks of leading others into a deeper understanding of just what illness is and how previously conceived lifelong illnesses can be reversed.

The next step is to be patient with the process and stay true to the regimen you have created for yourself according to these guidelines. During this time, make it a daily practice to envision what your life looks like after the healing process is completed. Trust it, reinforce it, and believe it whole-heartedly to be true. Your thoughts determine your reality.